Education, Disordered Eating and Obesity Discourse

Eating less, exercising more and losing weight seem the obvious solution for the oncoming 'obesity epidemic'. Rarely, however, is thought given to how these messages are interpreted and whether they are, in fact, inherently healthy.

Education, Disordered Eating and Obesity Discourse investigates how 'body-centred talk' about weight, fat, food and exercise is recycled in schools, enters educational processes and impacts on the identities and health of young people. Drawing on the experiences of young women who have developed eating disorders and research on international school curricula and the media, the authors challenge the veracity, substance and merits of contemporary 'obesity discourse'. By concentrating on previously unexplored aspects of the debate around weight and health, it is revealed how well-meaning advice can propel some children towards behaviour that seriously damages their health.

This book is not only about 'eating disorders' and the people affected but the effects of obesity discourse on everyone's health as it enters public policy, educational practice and the cultural fabric of our lives. It provides both a radical and challenging perspective on health issues that will interest students, teachers, doctors, health professionals and researchers concerned with obesity and weight issues.

John Evans is Professor of Sociology of Education and Physical Education in the School of Sport and Exercise Sciences, Loughborough University, UK.

Emma Rich is Lecturer in The Body and Physical Culture in the School of Sport and Exercise Sciences, Loughborough University, UK.

Brian Davies is Emeritus Professor of Education at Cardiff University, UK.

Rachel Allwood is a doctoral research student in the School of Sport and Exercise Sciences, Loughborough University, UK.

Education, Disordered Eating and Obesity Discourse

Fat fabrications

**John Evans, Emma Rich,
Brian Davies and Rachel Allwood**

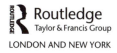

Routledge
Taylor & Francis Group

LONDON AND NEW YORK

First published 2008 by Routledge
2 Park Square, Milton Park, Abingdon, Oxon OX14 4RN

Simultaneously published in the USA and Canada
by Routledge
270 Madison Avenue, New York, NY 10016

Routledge is an imprint of the Taylor & Francis Group, an informa business

Typeset in Times by
Keystroke, 28 High Street, Tettenhall, Wolverhampton
Printed and bound in Great Britain by
CPI Antony Rowe, Chippenham, Wiltshire

British Library Cataloguing in Publication Data
A catalogue record for this book is available from the British Library

Library of Congress Cataloging in Publication Data
Education, disordered eating and obesity discourse : fat fabrications /
John Evans . . . [et al.].
    p. ; cm.
1. Obesity in children–Prevention–Social aspects. 2. Eating disorders in
children–Social aspects. 3. Health education. 4. English language–Discourse
analysis. I. Evans, John, 1952 Oct. 16–
[DNLM: 1. Obesity. 2. Adolescent. 3. Eating Disorders. 4. Health Education.
5. Health Policy. 6. Social Environment. WD 210 E24 2008]

RJ399.C6E383 2008
362.198'92398–dc22
                                  2007048093

ISBN10: 0–415–41894–1 (hbk)
ISBN10: 0–415–41895–X (pbk)
ISBN10: 0–203–92671–4 (ebk)

ISBN13: 978–0–415–41894–2 (hbk)
ISBN13: 978–0–415–41895–9 (pbk)
ISBN13: 978–0–203–92671–0 (ebk)

'Y Gwir yn Erbyn y Byd'

Contents

Foreword

Body pedagogics, society and schooling

Chris Shilling

Introduction

The manner in which bodies are marked, modified, nourished, educated and experienced has long been considered key to understanding the central characteristics of a society's culture. Anthropologists have demonstrated this in their analyses of how ritual feasting, fasting, tattooing and scarification reflect status differences and serve as corporeal boundaries between tribal groups (Douglas, 1970). Sociologists have also been interested in how such corporeal processes can be interpreted as actual indicators of social reproduction and change (Shilling, 2008). Emile Durkheim (1995 [1912]), for example, argued that the emotional effervescence generated when embodied subjects met in the presence of 'the sacred' shaped how people related to their own bodies and affected the development of the social body. Writing from a contrasting theoretical perspective, Max Weber's (1991 [1904–5]) explorations into the Protestant ethic identified the development of a historically distinctive *habitus* as a corporeal foundation for the advance of rational capitalism.

Studies such as these have been interpreted in various ways (e.g., as investigations into social symbolism, as demonstrations of the determining power of social facts, or as evaluations of meaningful social action), but what they have in common is an explication of the social importance of what we might refer to as the cultural *body pedagogics* characteristic of a society. This shared interest in body pedagogics is based on the recognition that culture is not just a matter of cognitive or symbolic knowledge but entails an education into socially sanctioned bodily techniques, dispositions and sensory orientations to the world (Mauss, 1973 [1934]). In seeking to explicate the full implications of this insight for both social groups and individuals, however, the study of body pedagogics goes beyond the simple but important recognition that 'bodies matter'. Instead, it highlights the reciprocal interactions that occur between embodied subjects and the collectivities in which they live via its concern with the primary pedagogic *means* through which a culture seeks to transmit its main corporeal techniques, skills, norms and beliefs, the *experiences* typically associated with acquiring or failing to acquire these attributes and the actual *embodied outcomes* resulting from this process. These corporeal outcomes provide the basis on which cultures and the societies in which they are based are subsequently either consolidated or challenged. Thus, Durkheim's depiction of body pedagogics centred on the ritual means of cultural reproduction, in which collective experiences tended to result in an intensification of shared ways of marking the body and a strengthening of social solidarity. In contrast, Weber focused on a Puritan body pedagogics, in which individualised engagements with the word of God constituted the means by which believers experienced their this-worldly lives as isolated and disenchanted. This experience resulted in a tendency for work to be viewed as a potential route to salvation; an outcome which provided a basis for social and economic transformation.

Classical sociologists such as Durkheim and Weber generally explored those forms of body pedagogics central to the inception and development of *industrial* society, or those minimal forms that could be associated with the consolidation of *any* social group. They could not be expected to anticipate the manner in which the body has, in recent decades, become quite such an obsession for governments and individuals. In order to explore this trend in more detail, it is worth turning to the work of Martin Heidegger who produced one of the most relevant and disturbing visions of the body pedagogics associated with the culture of advanced technological society in the West, and provides us with a prescient warning about its consequences.

The body pedagogics of technological culture

According to Heidegger (1993 [1954]), the essence of technological culture (as it has developed in the West) involves an instrumental rationalism of total mastery over nature. This serves to 'enframe' nature by calling upon the environment to be 'immediately on hand' as a 'standing reserve' forced to yield its properties and potential to *any* efficiency-based demand placed upon it. Consequently, the defining property of advanced technological culture is an insistence on domination and control *irrespective* of the properties of the material with which it is involved, something that reaches a point where *people* themselves are regarded as a standing-reserve for the demands of a system that prioritises production over all else. What is tragic about this situation is that it is unrecognised by the majority of those subject to it: individuals are so used to regarding the world through the prism of rational instrumentalism that they fail to see that they have become the object of this logic (Heidegger, 1993 [1954]: 320, 329, 333).

Heidegger did not examine in detail the processes through which the technological enframing of the body is initiated and sustained (Heidegger, 1979) but it is possible to summarise the body pedagogics associated with this development (Shilling and Mellor, 2007). In contrast to Weber's Puritans (for whom work was an *ethical vocation*), the demands of work as a pervasive, purely instrumental activity in the sphere of production and consumption constitute the dominant means by which technological culture is transmitted. Here, our bodily selves are increasingly subject to performative expectations in the labour market and also in a consumer culture centred on visions of physical perfection. The characteristic experience associated with this instrumental orientation towards life is that the body becomes *objectified* as an absent–present raw material that we are responsible for controlling in line with external standards (rather than as the vehicle of our sensuous and creative being-in-the-world). Finally, the outcome of these technological body pedagogics is that the embodied subject is either positioned as a *standing reserve* for the demands of productivity or is stigmatised and viewed as morally suspect. The precise manner in which this 'enframing' of the body proceeds varies across particular institutions, but contemporary approaches to *health* exemplify much about how this culture is being embodied in the present era.

Health, performativity and the pursuit of perfection

In the past, health and sickness have been conceptualised as intimately connected. This is evident in Susan Sontag's (1991: 3) suggestion that we all hold dual passports to 'the kingdom of the well' and 'the kingdom of the sick' and in Talcott Parsons' (1991 [1951]) enormously influential depiction of the 'sick role'. The latter constituted a temporary role – into which all may be admitted, at some time in their lives, with the permission of doctors – and marked societal recognition of the impermanence of robust health. As the twentieth century came to a close, however, people faced growing pressure to maintain their health as an important part of what was involved in conforming to the values of an increasingly competitive society. Emerging initially alongside the sick role, and then rising to a position of increasing dominance over it, was the 'health role' (Frank, 1991).

The health role differs from the sick role in terms of its emphasis on the *maximisation* of people's productive capacities and performances and on the importance accorded to *preventing* the experience of illness. The significance accorded to these activities by technological culture is clear. As Parsons (1978: 69) noted, modern societies are concerned with health as it enables us to perform a 'wide range of functions' *in relation to* the needs and demands of the social system. In this context, while the sick role invests the ill with a responsibility for seeking out medical help and following professional advice in order to return to their social roles, the health role places on people the responsibility for *not getting ill or impaired in the first place*. In accordance with the body pedagogics of technological culture it is a role that requires individuals to work on their own bodies – in a constant vigil against frailty and ill health – so that their bodies can work, at their most productive level, within society.

The health role has become institutionalised at the level of the nation state through the medicalised surveillance of populations (Foucault, 1973). Here, the premise is that productive health is threatened by a variety of behavioural and environmental risk factors that require constant monitoring and regular intervention, and that the government creates the context in which individuals are encouraged to maintain their performative capacity. Risk assessments are regularly conducted in workplaces, for example, and have resulted in such measures as bans on smoking and the drug testing of employees (Jackson, 1995), while the World Health Organisation as well as individual governments have set targets and implemented strategies designed to reduce accidents in the home and workplace and on the roads (Green, 1995). A further manifestation of the institutionalisation of the health role is apparent in the increasing incidence with which health services and health insurance companies reward and penalise their clients (through the scope of coverage they offer and the premiums they charge) for their lifestyle. Those who are classified as overweight, or who smoke or drink 'excessive' quantities of alcohol, face higher premiums and the possibility of being prevented from undergoing certain operations and procedures (Frank, 1991: 209).

There are partial historical antecedents to the health role but the extent of its concern with productive capacity is unprecedented. It is no longer just temporary or chronic illness preventing people from discharging their usual social roles that is deemed problematic but *anything* that interferes with individuals feeling, looking and being at their best in a social milieu in which health is prized, expected and, increasingly, demanded as a marker of productive efficiency. In order that individuals can discharge their responsibility in relation to the health role, the main 'right' they have involves access to a seemingly ever expanding quantity of health-related products and services. From fitness programmes, to diet products, to food supplements, to cholesterol-lowering drugs, the market for orthodox and alternative health-enhancing products is matched by increased information about health (Cant and Sharma, 2000: 430). Foods, drinks and other consumables come packaged with risk calculations and warnings on the assumption that 'knowledge about the dangers of certain lifestyle activities will result in their avoidance' (Lupton, 1994; Gabe, 1995: 2).

The health role has been assessed as implicating contemporary individuals within a new and more demanding mechanism of social control which 'banishes' illness and disability 'from everyday life' and associates infirmity 'with a lack of individual strength' (Kleinman, 1992: 205). Against this background, there is now no excuse for failing to pursue the development of a 'culturally approved' body. In these circumstances, it is easy for the chronically ill or impaired to 'feel that they are culturally illegitimate, unaccepted in the wider society' (*ibid.*). More worrying still is the potential the health role has for making *everyone* feel inadequate and even deviant. As *Education, Disordered Eating and Obesity Discourse* demonstrates, this can have particularly detrimental consequences for younger members of society.

Education, obesity and the health role

As the health role has become increasingly pervasive over the last few decades one of its most visible manifestations has been the concern accorded to the 'obesity epidemic' that is apparently sweeping through the affluent world and causing untold damage to the future of today's children (Gard and Wright, 2005). Governments, health organisations, sports agencies and the media have joined together to fight this spectre and one of the principal means through which they have chosen to do so involves education. Information regarding the success or otherwise of such educational campaigns remains scarce, but even rarer are analyses which help us to understand how these messages are operationalised within the most important educational arena of all – the school. It is here that *Education, Disordered Eating and Obesity Discourse* comes into its own as a unique contribution to our understanding.

John Evans, Emma Rich, Brian Davies and Rachel Allwood are highly critical of the 'science' behind the current obsession with obesity, and do an excellent job in revealing how 'obesity' cannot be considered a given but is a cultural and historical variable measured contemporarily by unreliable devices such as the Body Mass Index (BMI). The prime aim of *Education, Disordered Eating and Obesity Discourse*, however, is to explore how the *messages* regarding obesity, weight, health and fatness that have become integral elements of the health role are *recontextualised* in schools and affect the lives of young people. No study has explored this aspect of educational body pedagogics before and the manner in which Evans, Rich, Davies and Allwood undertake this task is groundbreaking. Their explorations proceed by revealing how an increasing number of educational issues, conversations, programmes and curricula are organised and operationalised on the basis of body-centred concerns with weight. They then identify two major problems with this in relation to the well-being of young people. The first is that the emphasis on weight and 'fitness' concerns in school overlooks or marginalises a series of other considerations that are important to young people yet are not provided with a place in this schema. Second, the effects of focusing on body and weight issues in a school environment already saturated by particular expectations regarding educational *achievement* can be potentially devastating.

Drawing on and extending Bernstein's analysis of the classification and framing of educational knowledge, Evans, Rich, Davies and Allwood capture the underlying principles which have governed this body-centric instantiation of the health role in schools through the notions 'performance codes' and 'perfection codes'. Their analysis traces in impressive detail how, of all the ways in which messages about health and well-being could be incorporated into a curriculum, knowledge about body management in schools is framed against the backdrop of a normative and highly partial vision of *corporeal perfection*. As they point out, 'healthy schools' are monitoring increasing areas of children's lives. Issues regarding healthy eating and drinking, personal hygiene, physical activity, acceptable body shape, slimming, relationship education and drug education are no longer 'private' matters but are required to be discussed and evaluated in the public realm of school. In this context corporeal perfection becomes a metric circulating in schools which can be, and is, used by children to classify themselves and their peers. Straying too far from physical perfection damages young people's standing with their peers: those considered obese have more difficulty making friends, and are more subject to bullying on the basis of stereotypes involving the equation that fatness = laziness + stupidity.

These perfection codes do not exist in a vaccum, but are operationalised in schools already committed to a culture of *performance*. As evident in the emphasis education systems place on tests, exams, team sports and individual athletic achievement, young people are already under significant pressure to succeed in assessments and competitions that will do much to determine their market value in and out of school. Introducing corporeal perfection codes to this environment has the potential to place a very substantial additional burden on them. As Evans, Rich, Davies and Allwood note, 'the body becomes just another way of achieving "performances" to meet the criteria of excellence, control and so on by which they feel they are judged by teachers or their peers'.

The manner in which young people respond to these expectations and pressures will obviously vary and the sociology of education has been adept at revealing how the culture of school is mediated and opposed by large sections of young people. What is perhaps distinctive about the manner in which the health role has been deployed in schools, however, is the degree of commensurability it has with wider cultural trends. The pursuit of bodily perfection has become so pervasive across society that the messages young people receive in school are reinforced outside of school in film, advertising, fashion and consumer culture more generally. The agents and technicians of 'bodywork' (Shilling, 1993: 118) populate our high streets and fill our television schedules in ever greater numbers. Cosmetic surgeons and personal trainers, as well as dietary and wellness gurus, shape the norms that affect how people view their bodies. In addition, the staple diet of prime-time reality television includes programmes that use chemical peels, cosmetic dentistry, liposuction, face-lifts and other forms of surgery in order to make their subjects appear thinner, younger and fit to take their place in a world in which (we are told) a prerequisite of success and happiness is *looking* healthy, trim and attractive. For those already predisposed to achieve at school, and especially for those young women having to cope with a culture that equates femininity with particularly restrictive body types, the cumulative pressure of these trends can be extremely troubling.

Evans, Rich, Davies and Allwood do not seek to provide a complete and exhaustive explanation for the behaviours of the young women in this study but they do succeed in revealing how the body pedagogics of schooling have changed in recent years and why we should be worried about these changes. Their analysis of the 'potent mix' of performance and perfection codes highlights the unintended consequences of contemporary forms of 'health education' in schools and suggests that these should come with their own health warning. *Education, Disordered Eating and Obesity Discourse* is not just a convincing critique of these developments, however; it has at its heart a concern to emphasise that things could be different. There is no necessity for us to embrace visions of health and the body which revolve around unrealistic and damaging notions of aesthetic perfection and limitless performativity, and it is worth concluding this foreword by highlighting the peculiar specificity of our current concern with physicality.

People have long undergone social pressures, physical ordeals and deprivations in line with cultural norms and it would be wrong to suggest that there has ever been a 'golden era' which provides us with a normative model against which to judge as wanting our contemporary approach to body matters. Early Christians and medieval ascetics engaged in fasting, cutting, marking and other forms of self-inflicted pain, for example, which bear certain comparison with the way in which

the body is disciplined and deprived in current discourse about slim, trim and productive bodies. What distinguishes these past behaviours from those associated with the current pursuit of physical perfection, however, is that they were linked to the search for religious truth and transcendental salvation (Bynum, 1987; Brown, 1988). The current concern with shape and appearance, in contrast, is linked to resolutely *this-worldly* standards of appearance and performativity.

Another characteristic of contemporary concerns with health as productive capacity is that they have no place for developed notions of human *well-being*. Again, this contrasts markedly with a number of other cultures. Contemporary Christian notions of well-being, for example, are predicated upon rituals of communion in which individuals symbolically incorporate into themselves the body of Christ and become incorporated into the body of the Church. Suffering, imperfection, frailty and our physical interdependence on others are central to, rather then excluded from, this notion of what it is to be an embodied being. Muslim notions of well-being also include an emphasis on physical interdependence with others of the same faith and impart a reassurance to those who live their lives in relation to the ethical standards laid down in the Qur'an and adhere to the 'five pillars' of Islam. The Taoist focus on cultivating a holistic sense of wellness by cultivating an equilibrium between the *yin* and *yang* energies of the body, and aligning these with those energies circulating outside of the individual, provides us with yet another contrast with the health role's concern with *productive capacity*. In the modern world, these religious cultures rarely *reject* technology, but they do engage with it on the basis of quite different sets of body pedagogics.

I mention these religious cultures here not to present them for endorsement, but to suggest that there is no inevitability or necessity for the current form of body pedagogics in schools. *Education, Disordered Eating and Obesity Discourse* shows us just how important a consideration of alternatives is. Evans, Rich, Davies and Allwood have produced an important critical study that should be required reading for all policy-makers, health professionals and teachers concerned about the well-being of young people. In providing young women with an opportunity to express their concerns about the body pedagogics they are subject to in schools, it illustrates the huge problems that can be caused by contemporary discourses about obesity.

Acknowledgements

This study would not have been possible without the support and cooperation of Dr Dee Dawson and staff at Rhodes Farm Clinic, The Ridgeway, London. We are particularly indebted to the young women at the clinic who spoke so eloquently of their experiences of education and schooling, and gave so generously of their time to take part in this study.

Many others, too numerous to mention, have also contributed to the development of this text and their advice, critique and contribution to the debate about obesity and health issues have been constant sources of enlightenment. In particular, we would like to thank Jan Wright, Michael Gard, Bethan Evans, Lisette Burrows, David Stensel, Rachel Sandford, Terry Mills, Geoff Whitty, Meg Maguire, Alan Bairner, Tom Page, Stephen Ball, Andy Miah, Andrew Sparkes, David Brown, Brett Smith, Cassandra Phoenix, Christie Halse, Hanelle Harjunen and especially Janet, Rhianedd and Ceryn Evans for their invaluable insight, good humour and enduring support.

Many thanks to Chris Shilling, Professor of Sociology at the University of Kent, for his Foreword and invaluable insight into the relationships between the body, society and schooling.

Some of the chapters in this book are revised, re-edited and expanded from previously published papers refined for the purposes of this text: Evans, J. (2003) Physical Education and Health: A Polemic, or, Let Them Eat Cake!, *European Physical Education Review*, 9: 87–103 (Sage Publications and North West Counties Physical Education Association); Evans, J., Rich, E. and Davies, B. (2004) The Emperor's New Clothes: Fat, Thin and Overweight: The Social Fabrication of Risk and Ill-health, *Journal of Teaching Physical Education*, 23, 4: 372–92 (Human Kinetics, Inc.); Evans, J., Rich, E. and Holroyd, R. (2004) Disordered Eating and Disordered Schooling: What Schools Do to Middle Class Girls, *British Journal of Sociology of Education*, 25, 2: 123–43 (Taylor & Francis Ltd); Evans, J., Rich, E., Davies, B. and Allwood, R. (2005) The Embodiment of Learning: What the Sociology of Education Doesn't Say about 'Risk' in Going to School, *International Studies in Sociology of Education*, 15, 2: 129–49 (Taylor & Francis Ltd); Evans, J., Rich, E., Allwood, R. and Davies, B. (2008) Body Pedagogies, P/policy, Health and Gender, *British Educational Research Journal*, 34, 3: 386–402; Rich, E. and Evans, J. (2005) 'Fat Ethics' – the Obesity Discourse and Body Politics, *Social Theory and Health*, 3, 4: 341–58 (Palgrave Macmillan). We are grateful to the publishers for permission to use this material.

Abbreviations and acronyms

Body Mass Index	BMI
Competency modes	CM
Department for Education and Skills	DfES
Department of Health	DoH
Diary data	(Dd)
Email correspondence	(Em)
Field notes	(Fn)
Focus groups	(Fg)
Health and physical education	HPE
Health education	HE
Informal conversations	(Ic)
Interviews	(In)
National Audit Office	NAO
National Child Measurement Programme	NCMP
National Curriculum	NC
National Curriculum Physical Education	NCPE
National Health Service	NHS
National Healthy Schools Programme	NHSP
National Institutes of Health (US)	NIH
Official recontextualising field	ORF
Pedagogic recontextualising field	PRF
Performance codes	PC
Performance modes	PM
Personal and social education	PSE
Personal, social and health education	PSHE
Personal, social, health and economic education	PSHEE
Physical education	PE
Physical education and health	PEH
Poster data	(Pd)
Totally pedagogised micro-societies	TPMS
Totally pedagogised society	TPS
United States Department of Health and Human Services	USDHHS
World Health Organisation	WHO

1 Introduction

The rise and rise of the child-saving movement

On 27 February 2007 the *Daily Mirror*, a popular British tabloid newspaper, reported the case of an 'overweight 8 year old, weighing 218 pounds', purportedly 'four times the weight of a "healthy" child of his age'. His mother feared she might lose custody of her son unless he lost weight, though she had been allowed to keep the boy after striking a deal with social workers to safeguard his welfare (Wagner, 2007). The child was in danger of being placed on the childcare register or even in care, measures usually applied to those suffering serious physical or mental abuse, simply, it seemed, for being too fat. Much of the popular media's accompanying narration of this event carried tropes now familiar in the reporting of 'obesity' issues, especially in the UK. Single-parent family, broken home, irresponsible parent, bad diet and lack of exercise were all traded in terms of a striking image of a 'morbidly obese' child, the embodied representation of being hopelessly inadequate, irresponsibly working class and all that young people are not supposed to be. That there can even be serious consideration of state intervention and regulation that contemplates removal of children from loving families is in itself deeply disturbing, raising issues of both social justice and personal rights. It also reflects the awesome authority that 'obesity discourse' and those who espouse it now possesses in defining how populations should think, act and 'read' the aetiology of illness and health. Similarly unencumbered by sufficient sensitivity either for the people concerned or possibly underlying 'truths', an earlier instance of such reporting had claimed that 'Child, 3, Dies from Being Too Fat' (*Daily Express*, 2004: 1), apparently echoing the indignation of politicians and members of an official obesity task force. Some weeks later it was severely castigated by the *British Medical Journal* (2004) and, ironically, the *Daily Mirror* (2004) for perpetrating nothing short of 'A BIG FAT LIE – "Obese" Girl, 3, had genetic disorder'.

The UK population is now told daily that it is 'too fat', 'overweight' or 'obese', that measures ought to be taken to make more people thin. 'The whole environment is conspiring against people. We are putting on weight even when we don't want to, because the forces ranged against us being slim are so powerful,' rail scientists involved in producing one such high-profile obesity report (Foresight, 2007; *Guardian Unlimited*, 2007: 2). It is argued that schools and teachers are ideally positioned to help address these putative growing health concerns through improved catering and spending more time on health education, fitness testing and sport. Such messages, repeated uncritically in the media, are not peculiar to the UK. In Hong Kong, China, Japan, Singapore, Australia, New Zealand, the USA, Canada, India and elsewhere similar news stories regularly appear, though not always with subtexts as insidious or blatant as 'fat equals working-class failure, thin equals virtue and middle-class success'. Populations are purportedly in the grip of a global 'obesity epidemic' (World Health Organisation, 1998), facing serious health problems and associated, imminent decline unless measures are taken to address them by central governments, health organisations, families and, most critically, individuals. The choices, it seems, are as easy to identify as they are to reconcile: either eat less and better, exercise more and lose weight; or get fat, become ill and die young. 'The first generation to die before their parents' has become the apparently irrefutable, yet frankly ludicrous, slogan echoing the fears of obesity task force experts, government spokespeople, health ideologues and their predominantly new middle-class audiences. New health curricula and fitness regimes have been introduced in abundance to schools in the UK, Australia, Asia, the USA and elsewhere to address the growing 'problem' and to ensure that pupils learn the benefits of healthy lifestyles, take enough exercise, eat better food and work harder at losing weight and becoming thin.

An avalanche of research reports, government papers and policies, health initiatives, books, journals and radio and television programmes have somewhat uncritically supported and endorsed such 'child-saving' views. The spectre of obesity has become the source of a global, multi-billion-pound industry of pub- lished diets, fat clubs, exercise centres, gyms, TV programmes, health foods/ vitamins and slimmers' magazines. But until recently little thought has tended to be given to how its messages are being 'read' by various sections of the population and whether, ironically, they may lead to health damage rather than heightened well-being. Some academics from across the natural and social science disciplines and medicine have begun to challenge the veracity, substance and merits of 'obesity discourse'. The form and content of contemporary talk about 'weight', as will be seen in Chapter 2, especially the adequacy and 'certainties' of knowledge produced within primary research fields, have now come under critical scrutiny: for example, by Monaghan (2005b) in Ireland, by Campos (2004) and Campos *et al*. (2006) in the USA and by Gard and Wright (2005) and Warin *et al*. (2008) in Australia. Many others have begun to document its expression in health policy and the school curriculum, including potentially damaging consequences for young people's body images and developing sense of self (e.g., Beckett, 2004; Burrows and Wright, 2004b; Evans *et al*., 2004; Johns, 2005; Halse, 2007; Treseder, 2007).

This book is grounded in this emerging literature and aims to contribute to the central critique of 'obesity discourse' and advance the debate on weight, education and health. Unlike much of the obesity literature which focuses on epidemiology, aetiology, measurement, costs and consequences for individuals and health systems, it will concentrate on aspects of the debate around weight and health that have not yet been addressed in any detail, by either proponents or opponents of 'obesity discourse'. In order to do this we will focus from a socio-cultural perspective on the way in which 'body-centred talk' around weight, fat, food and exercise is 'recontextualised' (delocated, relocated and refocused in schools within and alongside other disourses; see Bernstein, 1990: 188) and has an impact upon the health and embodied subjectivities of young people. It will pose, among several others, one question that may be unpalatable to many proponents of obesity discourse: 'Is obesity discourse and the health curriculum, and other initiatives produced, good for children's health and well-being?' In doing so, we propose to draw together themes and issues in the recent literature which include critiques of obesity discourse (e.g., Gard and Wright, 2005), studies of body image (e.g., Grogan, 1999; Frost, 2001), eating disorders (e.g., Hepworth, 1999; Malson, 1998) and educational practices (e.g., Evans *et al.*, 2004a; Tate, 2000) in novel and innovative ways. Our interest is not in trading claim with counter-claim but in how particular narratives around health and obesity come to be recognised as 'truths' and how these may influence how children and young people perceive themselves and are perceived by others, both in and out of school. We believe that it is time to consider more reflectively what claims and what practices can be made in this field, while demonstrating how dominant health discourses legitimate and endorse particular embodied actions and subjectivities.

Over a period of five years our research (see Appendix) has centred on the lives of some forty young women who were suffering from anorexia nervosa or bulimia nervosa involving 'weight loss' usually referred to as eating disorders (ED).[1] We prefer to use the term 'disordered eating' to describe their 'condition' because this both broadens and problematises our thinking on the nature ('aetiology', 'antecedents') and 'effects' of EDs. It also enables us to capture the different forms of control that these young women exercised over diet and to signal more widely that disordered relationships with food and associated exercise regimes are being displayed increasingly by individuals, who may not be medically classified as having an ED, as they engage in behaviours around them that potentially damage their health.[2] These young women are given a central role in how we explore features of obesity discourse as they reflect on their experiences of mainstream school and 'disordered eating'. All were full-time residents for a period usually lasting two to four weeks at a centre in England specialising in the treatment of such conditions, having been referred by general practitioners, child psychiatrists or paediatricians. Their costs were met either by the National Health Service (NHS) or by private means, usually provided by their families. At the time of study no males were resident at the centre. As participants in our research, they were asked to record and reflect on their experiences of mainstream schooling and how it may have influenced the development of their disordered eating. We place their experiences alongside research carried out on schools' health curricula to help document how obesity discourse, 'manufactured' in bioscience and recontextualised in the media, intersects with other factors within them, in families and among friends to propel some children towards behaviour that seriously damages their health and well-being. The actions and views of these young people who have taken 'disordered eating' to an extreme throw into sharp relief aspects of schooling, culture and society that are problematic for many other children and young people, not just 'the vulnerable few'. In this way, the book is not simply about 'eating disorders' and those affected by them but about the potential effects on everyone's health of obesity discourse as it enters public policy, educational practice and the cultural fabric of our lives. It is aimed with serious academic purpose at students, teachers, doctors, health educators, health professionals and researchers concerned with obesity and weight issues, offering theoretically informed critique of obesity discourse and health policies and their educational implications. We believe it is equally important to make each issue accessible to a wider readership by bringing alive issues through the voices of the young people who revealed to us how obesity discourse entered into and became part of their lives.

How we conceptualise recent developments in culture, health and obesity discourse and their translation into education policy and practice will have a bearing on how we interpret the stories that young people tell about their school experiences and how we read the aetiology of their concerns. We draw connections between what, for some young people, are deeply personal, private and emotionally loaded 'troubles' and very public, global health concerns (Mills, 1959), examining sceptically the notion of value-free discourse in this area of study in the context of the claims of bioscience, health experts and politicians, as well as our own assertions. In Chapter 2 we draw attention to our theoretical framework and personal priorities. We introduce the key concepts and perspectives used to research the voices of the young people that will be heard throughout these pages, such as 'obesity discourse', 'pedagogic discourse' and 'body pedagogies', as simple, heuristic devices for better understanding the social relations and networks relating to 'health' and behaviours defined as 'disordered'. We hope that their juxtaposition offers a more complex model than is currently found in the literature for understanding disordered eating and wider health issues, and takes us beyond thinking of 'eating disorders' as merely gendered reflections of society's obsession with particular corporeal ideas concerning 'the slender body'. The subtext of this chapter is that debate relating to the aetiology and treatment of weight gain and obesity cannot be dislocated from issues around 'underweight', weight loss, social class and gender and that a great deal might be learned about 'obesity' and the way it is treated in obesity discourse from the lives of people who 'decide' to become dangerously thin. In broaching these issues, however, we argue that before engaging with how 'health' enters the lived experience and becomes part of the embodied consciousness of young people we need to consider how it is constructed as a form of pedagogic discourse by bioscience and circulated both in popular culture through various media forms, including TV, magazines and websites, and in formal education.

In Chapters 3 and 4 we foreground how particular forms of health knowledge are constructed as either 'sacred' (abstract, legitimate, truthful, unambiguous, objective, 'good') or 'profane' (concrete/contaminated, illegitimate, equivocal, subjective, popular, 'bad') by centring attention on various components of obesity discourse. Chapter 3 focuses on its *instructional* components and codes[3] that not only define what 'health' is but what skills and competencies are required of populations to achieve it. We consider what is meant by 'overweight', 'obese' and 'fat' and how these rather slippery concepts dominate medical and popular thinking on bodily health, shape and mortality, and whose interests they serve. We pay particular attention to the way in which Body Mass Index (BMI) has become the primary tool not only for measuring but for regulating people's thinking and actions on body size, shape and health. It has assumed immense power and significance as a measurement tool within science, medicine and contemporary health education policy and practice. Building on the work of Campos (2004), Gard and Wright (2005) and Evans *et al.* (2004a), we examine BMI as a 'social construction', interrogate its fault-lines and falsehoods and note the fabrications conjured up in its name. When applied uncritically by health professionals, doctors, health workers and teachers, in and outside schools, the potentially damaging effects of BMI measurement and its accompanying rationales are amply illustrated by the young people who spoke to us.

Chapter 4 centres on the *regulative* components of health discourse which, together with the instructional, form the pedagogic discourse and practices pervasive in UK schools. Here our analysis differs from previous critiques of obesity discourse (Gard and Wright, 2001; Campos, 2004). With Wright and Harwood (2008), we offer a wider assessment of the regulative functions of bio-pedagogies in culture and explore how regulative and instructional discourse shapes specific body pedagogies in schools and out. We also explore the ethical dimensions of current health policy and practice and the guidelines around weight issues to which they give rise, documenting how contemporary representations of obesity not only provide medical 'facts' but create social meanings which influence how schoolchildren as embodied subjects are to be viewed and assessed. Seldom in medical debates about obesity do we find discussion of the way in which morally loaded representations of the body affect individuals' sense of self and embodied identity. A variety of moralistic approaches to the body and health are present in obesity discourse but are rarely made available for public scrutiny. Offering a further advance on critiques of obesity discourse, we illustrate how 'thinness' has been cultivated as a universal value, leading to ethically dubious health policies which can have negative impacts on the social identities and lives of people, as well as wider cultural understandings of health, weight and 'fat'.

Throughout Chapters 1 to 5 we emphasise that pedagogical activity can no longer be thought of as confined to schooling. It also occurs in various other socio-political and cultural sites, such as families, schools, churches, mosques and doctors' surgeries, in which work on the body occurs. Obesity discourses do not reach straightforwardly into the lives of young people and certainly not only through formal educational practices. Chapter 5 examines how they circulate as part of popular culture in wider society through the media and websites as a form of 'popular pedagogy' before finding their way into schools both through official 'Policies' and informal 'policy' initiatives. Obesity discourse as popular pedagogy is formed as part of a relentless cycle of policy and spin, spin and policy, generating initiatives driven by the moral panic that has come to characterise the making of 'relevant' political agendas and social and educational policies intended to address them. We address ways in which 'obesity discourse', produced and manufactured in fields of primary research, becomes recontextualised by the media (Miah and Rich, 2008) in the UK and elsewhere. With specific reference to the James Spurlock film *Super Size Me* and several Jamie Oliver TV series (*JOTVS*), clear illustration of dramatic, sometimes even hysterical, media reporting of the 'obesity crisis' is offered to show how 'fat and overweight' people are represented publicly in ways that would not be acceptable were the reference point any other condition of 'ill health'. Normal, healthy, 'overweight' and 'fat' people and their families are routinely pathologised and defined as being 'at risk' to themselves, 'a risk' to society, and irresponsibly 'ill'. Such narratives tend to be classed, gendered and racialised, effectively invoking particular forms of citizenship in which individuals are implored to look after not only their own but the nation's health in what Halse (2007) calls 'bio citizenship'. In effect, they endorse the labelling and stereotyping of overweight and fat people that we find reported in schools. Here the voices of young people in our study illustrate the deep significance of media as forms of popular pedagogy. They tend to frame our thinking about our bodies and health in which 'overweight', 'fat' and 'obese' are rarely thought of as conditions of health. Instead, they are interpreted as inherently 'bad things', essentially products of individuals' or families' irresponsible behaviour, independent of the actions of governments and organisations or cultural and class conditions. It can be little wonder that the young women in our study come to regard their extreme behaviours as exemplary, if regrettable, reflections of the highest health ideals, as we will see later.

Media images do not, however, 'cause' weight loss and weight gain, though they are an important element in complex and multi-layered processes underpinning disordered relationships with food, exercise and health. Popular culture intersects with formal education and the practices of teachers in schools to impact upon the lives of young people. Chapter 6 highlights the distinctive features of contemporary health pedagogy. Its somewhat inescapable presence across all aspects of school life has come to differ markedly from previous physical education (PE) or health and physical education (HPE), subject-based, health-promotion strategies confined to the timetable. Life in schools tends to be increasingly driven by a culture of individualism, one of whose manipulating mantras is 'obesity discourse'. It has become extraordinarily difficult for pupils to avoid the pressures of performative culture, to escape the gaze of the many who now feel that they are either formally or informally 'authorised' by public health discourse to monitor and *assess* their state of health, essentially with reference to shape and weight. Within this culture it is difficult for pupils to locate times and spaces where they can 'be themselves' and feel that they can safely reveal what and who they 'really' are and want to be. Schools, we argue, have become totally pedagogised micro-societies (TPMS) in which health education is everywhere and everyone's concern (see Chapter 6). The effects of obesity discourse multiply in such contexts as they are reflected in official pedagogy and the overt and hidden curricula of schools. We make reference to recent, major initiatives to improve the diet, exercise and health of young people in the wake of the 'obesity crisis', such as Jamie Oliver's initiative on school dinners in the UK and the introduction of fitness testing regimes, health components of personal, social and health and physical education curricula and 'fat camps' in the UK, USA, Australia and elsewhere. They reproduce, reflect and are constrained by the main motifs of obesity discourse in a performative culture, with health and education policies assuming similar ideational guises. Here young people speak of how 'health education', so configured, contributed, if unintentionally and indirectly, to their ill health, pointing to ways in which schools might avoid contributing to young people's ill health.

In Chapter 7 we begin to explore how 'obesity discourse' intersects with other powerful and dominant currents, especially neo-liberalism, within formal education. Our concern in this chapter is to highlight certain social class dimensions of contemporary health policy and how they are mediated through dominant education ideologies and practices infused with what we will later refer to as 'performance' and 'perfection' codes (Evans and Davies, 2004) which regulate, among other things, pupils' relationships to knowledge, authority and their own and others' bodies. Such codes are highly volatile, emphasising competition and manifest display of appropriate body (corporeal) behaviours over many aspects and areas of school life. Obesity discourse and the practices it engenders can be read as a reflection of (White) middle-class values and legitimisation of a new, child-saving crusade addressing the under-socialised, pathological and corporeally misbehaved. However, it does not follow that it benefits all middle-class children in the process, even though they are inevitably counter-positioned discursively as having 'correct' morality, respectability and corporeality. Here, again, the voices of the young people illustrate the pervasiveness of these codes in formal education, how they are sometimes reinforced and endorsed by parents and peers and how seriously damaging they have been to their psychological and physical health.

All this, of course, is to confirm that learning as a cognitive process is always both 'embodied' and *affectively* loaded, so that how and what we learn and what endures in our experience of schooling are often determined by the extent to which they have tapped into and touched us at an emotional level, leaving some enriched and others, perhaps, emotionally scarred. Chapter 8 highlights the complexity and importance of 'emotions' or, more particularly, the affective dimensions of corporeality and 'desire' in teaching and learning in terms of the immense 'risks' involved, especially to some young women, in displaying them within performative school cultures. We foreground how young people *feel* when they hear and see that they are not the right shape, size and weight, and how and where they learn 'appropriate responses' to the pressures of being constantly 'in the gaze' of professionals and peers surveying their behaviour around food, weight, shape and exercise, reading their 'disorder' through the lens of performativity. Critically, we begin to explore how these experiences are interpolated by what we refer to as the *corporeal device*, embodied and *gendered*, and convey the 'real', felt, emotional implications of obesity discourse in young people's lives. Throughout these chapters, with reference to these young women, we also emphasise that 'weight loss' and 'weight gain' are learned processes involving rational 'choices' and 'emotional costs', critical incidents, phases and 'coping strategies' in contexts – not always of individuals' making – that cannot be avoided and are damaging to health.

Having done this, we ask whether it could be otherwise. Are there other discourses offering alternative versions of health that we might draw on to warrant more inclusive and less harmful body pedagogies in and outside schools? If so, how are we to assess them reflectively as 'counter science' and their attendant truth claims? With such questions in mind, Chapter 9 provides conceptual tools for 'reading' obesity and alternative discourses critically, underlining the importance of grounding health practices and initiatives in the material circumstances of people's lives. It does this by turning to a variety of perspectives which lie submerged beneath dominant discourses within nutrition, physiology, epidemiology, health science and medicine that offer alternative, more cautious and circumspect readings of 'weight' and 'health' than is evident in much 'mainstream' obesity literature produced both internationally – for example, by the World Health Organisation – and by central governments. We argue that unless policy-makers and educationalists embrace some of these 'alternative perspectives', along with acceptance that social class, ethnicity and other cultural and structural conditions influence people's choices and opportunities to be healthy, in their analyses of health behaviour, they are unlikely to create policies and practices that have a lasting and positive impact on people's lives.

According to Stephen Ball (2007a: 184), conclusions are 'modernist conventions which typically represent knowledge in a particularly authoritative way'. We, like him, see what we have done here as no more than to offer 'a set of starting points, an outline of methodological and conceptual possibilities', in our case for rethinking health and pedagogical issues, rather than as conclusive. Though, as Ball confesses, much of what tends to follow such cautionary notes 'does not exactly sound tentative'; our 'conclusions' in Chapter 10, like Ball's, are offered as uncertain, cautionary tales, aimed at raising critical awareness rather than offering prescriptions for health education practice in society and schools. Our position is driven, not least, by the limitations of the research to which we refer. It is to be acknowledged that we speak of educational practice in schools 'second hand', through the reflections of the young women in our study. And while the veracity and authenticity of their voices are not in question, their insights point towards the need for further research before we may generalise from what they have to say. Furthermore, despite our claim to be voicing the experiences of the young people in our study, our authorial voices dominate this text even while being, hopefully, grounded in their reflections on the turmoil, troubles and challenges of their lives.

Finally, with reference to what we identify as the four primary fat fabrications of obesity discourse, we ask what can health professionals learn about social and psychological aspects of obesity and weight gain from young people recovering from excessive dieting, exercise and weight loss, and what is to be learned from listening to their accounts of the processes, obstacles and support structures with which they have had to engage when trying to regain weight, rebuild positive relationships with food and exercise, and become 'healthy' within cultures that repeatedly press them towards becoming dangerously thin? We suggest that by foregrounding the socio-cultural and educational complexity of behavioural change we learn that class and culture, rather than weight and exercise, should be our central political and pedagogical concerns. We also learn of the futility of single-solution remedies to health problems, for example, of engaging in media literacy programmes, or crash diets, or exercise regimes while disregarding class and culture. While highlighting the extended timescales involved in changing lifestyles and attitudes towards exercise, food and weight, we point to the inherent limitations and health dangers of some of these and other initiatives. They constitute largely wasted motion without political action addressing the systemic excesses of performative culture in formal education.

The voices of young people, their stories and some of the incidents marking their 'illness' and recoveries make a profound contribution to our understanding of and possible answers to contemporary health concerns. Disordered eating may have very little to do with either eating or weight and everything to do with social relations involving power and control in which achieving recognition and a sense of authenticity, within and outside schools, can seem and feel like impossible ideals. We advocate a critical perspective on contemporary discourse, imploring readers to consider the implications of our analyses not just for the school curriculum but for the work of all those in health settings. How should concerns with size and weight figure, if at all, in health discourse and practice? Rejecting the main tenets of obesity discourse, as we surely must, what educational and empirical choices are we left with, what dilemmas and decisions have we to address? Can 'health' be reconceptualised, perhaps salutogenically (see Antonovosky, 1996), as a culturally grounded, social process in which weight and shape are as irrelevant to any assessment of its achievement as our attire and the colour of our skin? What body pedagogic, corporeality and ethic would this enterprise entail?

2 Body pedagogies, obesity discourse and disordered eating

Whose fat is it anyway?

> In effect, to find someone biologically or cognitively impaired constitutes what James Holstein and Jaber Gubrium (2000) call a 'collaborative accomplishment'. It is an accomplishment of particular professional groups, working with particular assumptions and values within a complicit culture.
>
> (Gergen and Gergen, 2003: 205)

One of the more remarkable features of contemporary popular culture may turn out to be how moral virtue became entangled with corporeal ideals. In the process countless numbers of ostensibly 'fit', sentient human beings of all shapes and sizes, who three to four decades ago would have gone about their daily business thinking that there was nothing very much wrong with their general well-being and health, give or take a few ailments, some nagging aches and pains, ageing and a bit of excess fat, have been discursively shifted into regarding themselves as being 'irresponsibly' unwell. This has occurred neither through any fault of their own nor through any 'real' experiential change in corporeal condition for, indeed, in terms of increasing longevity, they are doing rather well, but because global agencies, such as the World Health Organisation (WHO), national central government bodies and countless 'expert' spokespeople have redefined their health status as such. Specifically, many are deemed either to have already succumbed to or to be in danger of becoming victims of the purported, virulent, global 'diseases' of 'overweight' or 'obesity' in a world where both popular and uncritical, academic presses warn them of an 'obesity time bomb' ticking away, especially in relation to young people's health (see Chapter 3). Rarely can so many people have been made to feel so bad about their bodies or their routine maintenance through eating, moving, exercising and so forth, with so little concern or sensitivity as to the potentially damaging effects of this discourse. Yet research evidence suggests that, although populations have become on average marginally heavier over recent years, outside of the extremes of 'underweight' and 'obese', neither of these 'conditions' alone constitutes much of a risk either to the well-being or to the health of populations or persons (see Campos *et al.*, 2006). Indeed, 'several large studies show improved survival in heart patients with a body mass index of between 30–35

– classed as clinically obese' and one leading consultant criticised doctors for simply 'extrapolating the advice from the young and the fit to the old and the ill' (Smith, 2007: 10). Others have highlighted the dangers of applying 'adult' conceptions of 'healthy eating' to children and young people without regard for their maturational needs (Evans, 2007).

That the 'obesity crisis', as it is now commonly known, is a powerful element in the way in which our 'health' is 'storied into existence' and an artefact of changing medical classifications of overweight and, by association, 'ill health', has been well documented in the academic press, albeit with little accompanying critical debate. For example, Moynihan (2007: n.p.) observed that:

> A new and expanded definition of childhood overweight and obesity expected later this year is causing concerns that many healthy children may be unnecessarily labelled as having a disease.
>
> A powerful 'expert committee' in the United States has tentatively decided to reclassify children who are currently called 'at risk of overweight' and refer to them in the future as 'overweight'. Those familiar with these definitions say that such a change could lead to a dramatic expansion of prevalence estimates, with 25% of American toddlers and almost 40% of children aged 6 to 11 years portrayed as having a medical condition called 'overweight and obese'.

Others, too, have noted that the largest recent increase in the number of obese persons in America occurred in 1998 when the National Institutes of Health (NIH) lowered their BMI threshold for overweight downward two points from 27 to 25. In effect, overnight an additional 50 million Americans became 'fat' simply as an artefact of changing BMI guidelines, not through any increase in body weight (Boero, 2007: 47). These tendencies are not peculiar to the USA but are traded internationally. In Boero's view, they are an integral part of the 'obesity epidemic' forming a new breed of 'postmodern epidemic' in which 'unevenly medicalized phenomena lacking a clear pathological basis get cast in the language and moral panic of "traditional" epidemics' (*ibid.*).

'Panics' are, of course, commonplace in popular culture, whether white sharks off Cornwall, bird flu in Barnsley or escaped boa constrictors in South Wales, as the seed corn of modern media reporting, the stuff of which newspapers are made. More often than not they are irrelevant and ephemeral, no more than passing flotsam on the surface routines of our lives and of little consequence to them. *Moral* panics are rather different, especially if they endure, speaking to our values and dispositions and seeking to change the way in which we lead our lives. While here we simply foreground the social purposes they serve in fostering and establishing new norms, in Chapter 5 we explore in greater detail ways in which such panics are nurtured in popular media representations of weight issues, enabling us to consider whose interests they maintain in terms of equity and inclusion in society and schools.

Chomsky (2005) argued that to establish a norm you 'have to do something', noting that not everyone has the capacity to create one. They need power – either significant, ideological/discursive power, for example, the authority of a particular science or medicine, or physical power (mighty armies) – to do so. The easiest way to establish a new norm – for example, the right to take children away from their parents for being 'too fat' or to make 'fat' a sin – is to select a completely defenceless target, such as the poor working classes or single-parent families, which can be easily overwhelmed or vilified without riposte. In order to do that credibly in the eyes of your own population, Chomsky notes that people have to be frightened, the defenceless target demonised and characterised as an impending threat to population survival, and so on. So the 'fat' and, by innuendo, poor people or the inadequate, middle- or working-class single-parent families that produce them, are represented as irresponsible monsters, threats to the social order because of their misuse or overuse of resources. This is a view that many in the population (those who are not fat) are now beginning to accept: 'The doctrine is pronounced, the norm is established, the population is driven into a panic and believes the fantastic threats to its existence, and is therefore willing to support intervention by force if necessary in its defence' (*ibid.*: 2–3). What is more, we are led to believe that 'we' (or the state on our behalf) are doing this selflessly and graciously, to protect the fat 'othered' from the danger and damage they represent to themselves.

The so-called 'obesity epidemic' offers an example *par excellence* of how such social norms are reinstated or formed. As we will see, health discourse is imbued with both instructional and regulative codes (see Chapters 3 and 4) that are intended both to regulate and to conserve a particular social order by drawing, or rather redrawing, boundaries around 'good' and 'bad' behaviour, defining what individuals and populations ideally 'ought' to be. In so doing, they invariably serve particular interests, marking out the already privileged (good) from the ever needy (bad), the deserving from the undeserving. There is nothing particularly unique or modern about such processes. Our 'health', in part, is always something that is, or has been storied into existence, and has never been value free. Thus it is ever fluid, always potentially redefined or readjusted by the advances and proclivities of the corporate interests of medicine, business and science, and prevailing values on the cultural terrain. With others in the sociology of health, we take the view that to understand 'health' we need to see it through analyses of the 'stories that circulate between bodies and signs' (Frank, 2006: 422), for example those purveyed by the 'official' agencies mentioned above and/or various media (including TV and film, as described in Chapter 5) and the embodied lived experience of young people in schools. In this view, 'health' for individuals and for communities:

> depends on which stories are heard, which are taken seriously and what sense is made of these stories [. . .] These stories are *subjectifiers*; they offer people terms of health subjectivity [. . .] bodily awareness is 'constantly being re-shaped by health as ideals and evaluations, sometimes a promise and sometimes a fear. [Health] is a conjunction of images from *outside* of bodies and feelings that emanate from what the stories represent as being *inside* bodies.
>
> (*Ibid.*)

Our concern is with how 'health' is storied into existence by 'obesity discourse' to become part of what Frank defines as the *'natural attitude'* towards it in individuals or populations (*ibid.*: 424; see Chapters 3 and 4). This is not to obfuscate or deny the body as a biological entity capable of becoming 'ill', 'feeling pain' and 'going wrong' from, among other things, being dangerously 'over-' or 'underweight' but to acknowledge the irreducibility of the body to either biology or culture. It announces that how we read both our own and others' bodies is neither arbitrary nor immutable and is always culturally defined.

Obesity discourse

Throughout this book we will refer to *obesity discourse* as a framework of thought, talk and action concerning the body in which 'weight' is privileged not only as a primary determinant but as a manifest index of well-being surpassing all antecedent and contingent dimensions of 'health'. Body Mass Index (BMI), a number calculated from individual weight and height,[1] is taken as a reliable indicator of body fatness for most people and is used to screen for weight categories that may lead to health problems. Lauded by government ministers and obesity spokespeople as the key to monitoring populations' health status, both inside and outside school, it is increasingly offered to the public as the means to monitor weight as symptomatic of current or potential 'health'. However, as we shall see in Chapter 3, BMI is rather less good at determining what can be said about health, particularly children's health, than some would have us believe. Yet, despite its acknowledged limitations, it continues to play a key role in the politicisation of health. The extent to which discourses 'produce what they name is a matter for empirical research' (Sayer, 2005: 79) and the narratives of obesity discourse can be shown to have offered 'stories', language and practices by which not only the 'public sector' but, literally, the 'public body', our individual 'body politics', is being regulated and reformed. Notwithstanding its fallibility, obesity discourse, with BMI among its indispensable tools, has been profoundly influential 'in providing possibilities for political thought and thus policy' (*ibid.*) in this case on health education in schools. As Frank (2006: 430) points out, people know themselves and each other by and through practices, and they know practices through stories: 'Stories perform the work of subjectification: they are subjectifiers, telling people who they ought to be, who they might like to be and who they can be.'

'Body pedagogics' and the medicalisation of our lives

The reclassification of populations globally as 'at risk' and in perpetual states of being 'potentially unwell' in what some refer to as the *medicalisation* of people's lives (Furedi, 2007) has been no accident any more than it has been conspiracy on the part of science or expression of political mischief or health educators' malicious intent. This process has owed as much to changing approaches in medicine to 'health' over the last forty years as to the way in which nation-states have increasingly sought to exercise authority and control over potentially recalcitrant populations, while simultaneously serving global capitalism's interests in generating surplus value, which rests on increasing consumption, even when dieting. In important ways in late twentieth-century medicine the quest for *cures* for ill health gave way to a search for its *causes*. This shift was driven by two very different specialities: 'new genetics' opened up possibilities of identifying abnormal genes in social diseases; and 'epidemiology' insisted that most common diseases, such as cancer, heart disease and diabetes, are caused by social factors connected to unhealthy lifestyles and are preventable by changing behaviour, such as switching diets, taking more exercise and reducing exposure to risk factors. Together, these approaches, especially when recontextualised through the ideologies and policies of neo-liberalism and free market economics, provide the basis for a radical shift from solving health problems through therapeutic measures to *intervention* – and the earlier the better – making the lives of children and young people and the places where they spend a good deal of their time, particularly among families and within schools, primary concerns of health and education policies.

At the same time in Western (and Westernised) societies coercive means of manipulating populations using explicit force and oppressive rule of law have given way to more subtle and less certain means of control involving a combination of mass surveillance and self-regulation which Foucault (1977, 1980) called 'disciplinary power'. Here, individuals and populations are ascribed responsibility for regulating and looking after themselves, though often according to criteria over which they have very little say or control, while, at the same time, being more or less relentlessly monitored in their capacity to do so, in some respects from cradle to grave (see Foresight, 2007: 63). As populations have grown and become more fluid and complex, nation-states have become 'more concerned about the management of life [**bio-power**] and the governing of populations' (Howson, 2004: 125), particularly in relation to health, disease, sexuality, welfare and education. Populations become objects of 'surveillance, analysis, intervention and correction across space and time' (Nettleton, 1992, quoted in Howson, 2004: 125). Bio-power, however: 'depends on technologies through which the state and its agencies can manage "the politics of life to shape the social to accord with the tasks and exigencies faced by the state"' (Hewitt, 1983: 225, quoted in Howson, 2004: 125). Foucault's reference 'to the knowledges, practices and norms that have been developed to regulate the quality of life of the population as bio-politics' indicates that the body becomes 'the raw material for this undertaking' (Howson, 2004: 126). Distinct physical spaces become locations in which people are monitored by those in authority who may observe them with minimum effort: 'Relations within such spaces are based on the observation of the many by the watchful eyes of the few, or on the "gaze" which judges as it observes and decides what fits – what is normal – and what does not' (Howson, 2004: 126). In such contexts new forms of normalising practices emerge in many sites of social practice through the exercise of what is now referred to as *body pedagogics* (Shilling, 2005, 2007), or *body pedagogies* (Evans and Davies, 2004, 2008) and their specific variants in schools. Such practices work as part of the bio-politics of contemporary Western cultures, steeped in obesity discourse (see Gard and Wright, 2005; Rich and Evans, 2005;

Campos, 2004). Elsewhere, Foucualt's (1979) concept of bio-power has also been instrumental in the development of the concept *bio-pedagogies* (Wright and Harwood, 2008) as a theoretical tool through which to examine the relationships between bio-power, obesity discourse and pedagogical practices. How bio-pedagogies are shaped to form the body pedagogies of popular culture and schools when infused with performance and perfection codes and the inherent meanings and principles of obesity discourse are at the forefront of our concerns.

Much of the discourse on obesity has focused on assumed relationships between childhood inactivity, young people's diets and claims about rapid rises in levels of 'overweight' and 'obesity'. It has generated something of a moral crusade in which children, perceived as under-socialised into correct ways of eating and exercising, become regarded as maladjusted or pathological, identified as a population 'at risk' of developing obesity and associated diseases and, therefore, in need of 'saving'. The WHO's 'global strategy on diet, physical activity and health, for example, recommends a variety of methods of control to curtail the "obesity problem", including instruction, surveillance and evaluation' (Groskopf, 2005: 41). Schools have been targeted as implementation sites for numerous initiatives geared towards getting children more active or 'thin' or changing their eating patterns. Such co-option of wider health concerns into health and education policies and their inclusion in pedagogical practice place young people under greater surveillance. They are also pressed to monitor their own bodies, not through coercion but by exposure to *knowledge* around 'obesity'-related risks and issues and instruction as to how to eat healthily, stay active and lose weight. As we shall make clear in Chapter 4, these instructional messages are deeply infused with a corporeal ethic, a socially regulative moral code.

In certain respects none of this is new but merely represents an extension, perhaps a new high point, of earlier, eighteenth-, nineteenth- and twentieth-century child-saving crusades (Platt, 1971: 97; see Chapter 10) which were also charac- terised by a 'rhetoric of legitimisation' built on 'traditional values and imagery', such as notions of 'the good life' uncontaminated by the pathologies of urban environments. They also borrowed images of pathology, disease and treatment from the medical profession, as well as 'from the tenets of Social Darwinism pessimistic views about the intractability of human nature and the innate defects of the working class'. To these were added ideas about the biological and environ- mental origins of 'crime' attributable to the 'positivist tradition in European criminology and to anti urban sentiments associated with the rural Protestant ethic' (*ibid.*: 96). In the early twentieth century, especially in the USA and the UK, there were policy shifts concerning delinquency 'from one emphasising its criminal nature to the "new humanism" which spoke of disease, illness, contagion, and the like', then, as now, representing essentially a shift from legal to medical emphasis, anticipating consequences that seem particularly redolent today:

> the emergence of a medical emphasis is of considerable significance, since it is a powerful rationale for organising social action in the most diverse behavioural aspects or our society. For example, the child savers were not

concerned merely with 'humanising' conditions under which children were treated by the criminal law. It was rather their aim to extend the scope of government control over a wide variety of personal misdeeds and to regulate potentially disruptive persons. The child-saver reforms were politically aimed at lower class behaviour and were instrumental in intimidating and controlling the poor.

(Ibid.: 102–3)

Our contention is that obesity discourse is a latter-day version of the 'child-saving' crusade, its goal being to rescue a child population 'at risk'. It is our task to articulate the changes in discourse that have occurred and their associated forms of control with the cultures and the principles of communication that govern policy and pedagogy in and outside schools. We seek to conceptualise how 'social facts' are encoded and embodied, how the instructional and regulative rules inherent in obesity discourse enter into and inhabit even the deep recesses of our minds.

Body pedagogies

Broaching these issues signals our shared interest in what Chris Shilling (2007: 13) has termed *body pedagogics*:

> the central pedagogic means through which a culture seeks to transmit its main corporeal techniques, skills, dispositions and beliefs, the embodied *experiences* typically associated with acquiring or failing to acquire these attributes, and the actual *embodied changes* resulting from this process.

We are also fundamentally concerned with cultural transmission, lived experience and embodied change. As Shilling (*ibid.*: 13–14) goes on to argue, however, the notion of body pedagogics:

> inevitably simplifies the myriad processes, complexities and variabilities involved in the transmission and development of cultures, but it nevertheless provides us with a useful ideal-typical and corporeally sensitive way of accessing some of its central elements involved in cultural reproduction and change.

While Shilling and Mellor (2007) seek to do so in addressing the body pedagogics of technology and religion, we focus attention on those of the media and the formal and informal practices of schools. We start from the view that while pedagogy constitutes 'any conscious activity by one person designed to enhance learning in another' (Watkins and Mortimore, 1999: 3) anywhere, no matter how apparently straightforward the event, 'both the what and how aspects of pedagogic discourse and its associated modalities of practice contain ideological elements that are never wholly utilitarian' (Bernstein, 1996, cited in Fitz *et al.*, 2005: 5). All pedagogies socialise, often as they simultaneously instruct and skill; all are value laden and help lay down the rules of belonging to a culture and class. All pedagogical activity is embodied (Shilling, 2005). *Body pedagogies* refer to any conscious activity taken by people, organisations or the state that are designed to enhance individuals' understandings of their own and others' corporeality. Occurring over multiple sites of practice, in and outside schools, they define the significance, value and potential of the body in time, place and space. Body pedagogics (Shilling, 2005, 2007) and their derivative body pedagogies produce particular, embodied subjectivities that are essentially corporeal orientations to self and others. These define whose and what bodies have status and value, constituting acts of inclusion and exclusion and carrying strong moral overtones. In obesity discourse, for example, individuals' character, value and sense of self come to be judged essentially in terms of 'weight', size or shape.

Body pedagogies construct particular social meanings which have an impact upon young people's identities in relation to both their health and to the academic performances they are expected to display and achieve. Indeed, the voices of the young people reported throughout this book highlight both the power and pervasiveness of bio-pedagogy, particularly in terms of defining and normalising particular dispositions and attitudes towards the body within a culture of 'performativity' where young people are subject to increasing pressures from exams, testing and other performance measures. As we see in Chapter 6, such systems of control have achieved ubiquity within a 'totally pedagogised society' (Bernstein, 2001). Here methods of evaluating, monitoring and surveying the body are encouraged across a range of contemporary cultural practices in schools, families, the popular media, new technologies and health organisations. Following Bernstein, we argue that schools have become totally pedagogised micro-societies (TPMS) in which concern for the shape and 'health' of 'the body' is no longer the preserve only of those subjects or areas of the curriculum historically concerned with body issues, such as physical education (PE), health education (HE) or personal and social education (PSE), but is now everyone's concern, everywhere, in classrooms, playgrounds, dining halls and corridors. No one – or, more accurately, 'no body' – escapes the evaluative gaze.

These are changes not only in the exercise of power but in the range and reach of authority and control into the lives of individuals and populations. In totally pedagogised societies 'disciplinary power', to use Foucault's glorious turn of phrase, is both

> absolutely indiscrete, since it is everywhere and always alert, since by every zone it leaves no zone of shade and constantly supervises the very individuals who are entrusted with the task of supervising; and absolutely 'discrete', for it functions permanently and largely in silence.
>
> (Foucault, 1977, in Lauder *et al.*, 2006: 127–8)

In this way, it is 'linked from the inside' not just of the organisation but the recesses of the subconscious 'to the economy' and to 'the aims of the mechanisms in which it is practised' as 'multiple, automatic and anonymous power: for although surveillance rests on individuals, its functioning is that of a network of relationships from top to bottom, but also to a certain extent from bottom to top and laterally' (*ibid.*: 128).

In Chapter 6 we further develop the notion of bio-power when encoded with specific ideals of *performance and perfection* in the totally pedagogised micro-societies (TPMS) that schools have become, with reference to recent health and education policies which shape body pedagogy and social relations.

A cautionary note: the complexity of social reproduction

As the voices of the young people in our research attest, while schools are primary sites of socialisation, complex processes of socio-cultural reproduction involve multiple sites of practice and multiple agencies, including churches, mosques and families in dynamic interaction with flows of 'popular pedagogies' in the media and on the web. However, most accounts of how health discourse is reproduced as pedagogy are overdetermined and rather limited versions of how obesity discourse 'normalises' and classifies individuals. The questions we seek to ask concern how power and control exercised in obesity and wider health discourse translate into principles of communication, specifically bio-pedagogy and body pedagogies. This is embedded in the even broader question of: 'how do these principles of communication differentially regulate forms of consciousness with respect to their reproduction *and* possibilities of change?' (Bernstein, 1996: 18; our emphasis). How do these processes occur in and outside schools? If our focus is upon formal education, it is necessary to shift the point of analysis implicit in health discourse from the school as a *relay* of class and cultural relations *external* to itself to study of the *medium* of transmission, the school's own voice – that is to say, the structure of pedagogy itself – as message systems both nurture particular forms of embodied consciousness and facilitate constraint *and* opportunity for resistance and change. As Bernstein (*ibid.*: 46–7) points out, pedagogic discourse is not a discourse in its own right but 'a principle by which other discourses are appropriated and brought into special relationships with each other'. He calls the discourse which creates specialised skills and their relationships to each other *instructional discourse* and the moral discourses which create order, relations and identity *regulative discourse*. He argues that instructional is always embedded in domi-nant, regulative discourse. 'The transmission of skills/understandings and the transmission of values always goes hand in hand. There is only one discourse' (*ibid.*: 47). Accepting this, we are obliged to interrogate 'obesity discourse' as comprising both instructional and regulative discourse, as generating and con-veying knowledge competencies and skills and moral codes, imperatives as to what and how 'the body' should be. As Bernstein stresses, all pedagogic discourse projects an interlocutor to whom the discourse is addressed. He refers to the interlocutor projected by pedagogic discourse as the *imaginary subject*. 'Subsumed within the imaginary subjects projected by "teachers" pedagogic discourse are ideological views about who children are and who they ought to become' (Ivinson and Duveen, 2006: 109). Furthermore, he refers to the medium as the voice of pedagogy (Bernstein, 1990: 190) that is constituted by the *pedagogic device*: 'a grammar for producing specialised messages, realizations, a grammar which regulates what it processes: a grammar which orders and positions and yet contains the potential of its own transformation'.

How does this bear on our study of young people and disordered eating? In Chapters 3 and 4 it leads us to interrogate how obesity discourse, constructed *outside* schools, helps form pedagogic discourse, foregrounding its instructional and regulative dimensions. These precede our attempts to understand how body pedagogies nurtured *inside* schools are infused with what we refer to in Chapters 6 and 7 as *performance and perfection codes* whose principles regulate but cannot 'determine' the embodied actions and positions of individuals. These chapters together highlight how the discursive intersection of instructional and moral imperatives forms pedagogic discourse, providing the principles that configure the body pedagogies and implicit pedagogic positions and identities that circulate in popular culture, the health curricula in schools and young people's responses to them.

We also set out to reveal the inherent ambiguities, ambivalences and contra- dictions in the knowledge base of obesity discourse and its attendant pedagogies. These are significant for two reasons. First, they tell us something about the nature and authority of 'truth narratives' and about how 'unhelpful facts' can either be obfuscated or ignored. Second, they are important because, as Bernstein (1996: 47) points out, in the recontexualisation of discourse between sites of practices – as, for example, in translation of government policy into school policy/initiatives – 'gaps open up, creating a space in which "ideology can play"' and individuals can read, interpret and recontextualise the received wisdoms or 'sacred' health knowledge that schools are meant to convey through the cognitive filters of their culture and class. As we see in subsequent chapters, young people are neither cultural dopes nor dupes. They act to recontextualise health knowledge critically through their own 'knower structures' (Maton, 2007), their personal, culturally encoded, affective understandings of their own and others' bodies and health, within the framework of the imperatives of health education policy and the performative cultures of their schools.

The corporeal device

Discourses are always inevitably mediated for young people through their agentic, material (flesh and blood, thinking and feeling) bodies, their actions and those of their peers, teachers and other adults. As a way of better articulating the *lived experiences* typically associated with acquiring the attributes required by obesity discourse and 'the actual embodied changes resulting from this process' (Shilling, 2007: 13), we are inclined, *pace* Bernstein, to talk of the *corporeal device*, to focus on the body as not just a discursive representation and relay of messages and power relations external *to itself* but as a voice *of itself*. As a material/physical conduit it has an internal grammar and syntax given by the intersection of biology, culture and the predilections of class, which regulate (facilitate and constrain) embodied action and consciousness, including the ways in which discursive messages (and all other social relations) are read and received. This concept privileges neither biology nor culture and endorses Frank's (2006: 433) view that neither 'the experience of embodied health nor the observation of signs of health circulating outside bodies has to trump the other as being the real point of origin. Instead each is understood as *making the other possible.*' This book will barely begin to touch the complexity of such relationships, though it will throw light on how the corporeal device finds expression as conscious and subconscious embodied action and is subjectified (given shape, form and definition as 'personality') in schools.

At one level, then, this book is an exercise in the sociology of knowledge. It is concerned with how health knowledge(s) produced in the primary field of knowledge production in science communities comes to be considered 'the thinkable' and 'sacred'; that is to say, official truth (reflected in 'Policy') as to what we ought to believe about the body and its capacity for health, fit to be purveyed in schools (see Figure 1). Indeed, like Monaghan (2005b), we will question whether the 'obesity debate' can be considered a debate at all. As it starts from a position of certainty and truth it leaves very little open to question. As we hold that 'truth' positions are not only possible and desirable but debatable within the field of health science (see Chapters 3 and 9), our analysis is intended to add insight into some of the enduring sociological questions about the production and interpretation of truth narratives in popular culture in relation to dominant discourses around health and risk. The mediations involved in this process between multiple sites of practice are relatively unexplored. Thus, at another level, this book is an exploration of embodied subjectivity as we trace how health knowledge(s) recontextualised within popular culture (through TV, websites and other media imagery; see Chapter 5) translate into education/health 'policies' (see Chapter 6) directed at the pedagogies of schools. These are ultimately mediated by the class and cultures of teachers and pupils, via the corporeal device. We suggest that, in this process, official health knowledge is separated or dislocated from everyday health knowledge – for example, about diet and exercise – which is reclassified and read as unhealthy or 'profane' (see Figure 1).

However, while drawing attention to the discursive content of health knowledge (see Chapter 3) we do not dwell either on the veracity of the statistics or the merits of the measurement tools, in particular the BMI, that have been used to inform education policy and populations that they are 'at risk' (see Gard and Wright, 2005). Our concern is to illustrate how a particularly *pathogenic* version of health has been constructed using the language of BMI as *the* 'right' way of thinking about health and the body, incorporated into policy and interpolated in the lives of young women via the practices of schools and wider popular culture. A pathogenic view of health starts 'from some view of normality where health equals normal' (Quennerstedt, 2007: 7) and focus falls on deviations from such so-called normality, as in 'morally correct' behavioural connotations around exercise and diet (Antonovsky, 1979, 1996). The notion that 'health' can be conceptualised or configured in quite different ways is written out of the narrative frame (see Chapter 9).

Media matters, popular pedagogy and performative culture

New forms of control are reflected in the voices of the young people in our study. Like the rest of us they can neither easily avoid the relentless messages of popular culture nor escape at least eleven years or 15,000 hours of their lives subject to technologies of self-regulation in formal education induced through policies and pedagogies relating to 'the body' and health. Though many young people are not easily seduced by it some are damaged in this process, their voices vividly illustrating the extent to which deeply felt, affectively loaded private issues and troubles around the body are inextricably tied to public cultures and global issues. As already mentioned 'disciplinary power' not only shapes and regulates the id and ego but links them to the economy and to the aims of the organisations in which they are 'practised' (Foucault, 1977). In subsequent chapters we highlight how the affective dimensions of formal education are governed by a 'performative culture' of individualism. We use the term 'performativity' throughout this book in two ways. First, following Butler (1990, 1994), it signals that our identities are always 'performed', that is to say brought into being as productive enactments or performances according to rules, expectations and resources available in particular social milieu. For example, we see that young people may perceive and understand 'health' as something to be displayed or 'performed' through appropriate actions, such as achieving the right body shape, size and weight or doing 'the correct' amount of exercise. Second, following Ball (2004a, 2007b: 692–3), we use it to refer to 'a culture and mode of regulation' (see Chapter 6), itself 'a system of measures, and indicators (signs) and sets of relationships', and, like him, we explore the 'fabrications' of the self that individuals are compelled to perpetrate to produce 'versions of themselves' within such contexts. As Butler (1990: 136) puts it: 'Such acts, gestures, enactments, generally construed, are "performative" in the sense that the essence or identity that they otherwise purport to express are fabrications manufactured and sustained through corporeal signs and other discursive means.' In a 'performative culture', schooling can seem insensitive and manipulative to young people endeavouring to adapt to, challenge or resist its requirements, or what may be experienced as its rather unattainable ideals. Their voices reveal that relationships between public health discourse, popular culture, formal education and disordered eating are rarely straightforward and never apolitical.

Increasing numbers of young people do report either dissatisfaction or disaffection with their bodies, and some, such as the girls in our study, go on to develop serious eating disorders. Anorexia nervosa does have the highest mortality rate among 'mental disorders' (van Hoeken *et al.*, 2003), though one barely gets to hear of the dangers of 'underweight' in the fat-focused, weight-loss cacophony of obesity discourse. But these facts do not imply that young people are passive readers of popular pedagogy or as easily swayed by media and celebrity cultures as the current frenzy around size-zero diets might have us believe. In our experience they are often far more 'savvy' than many of the adult 'experts' and academics inclined to pass judgement on their behaviour relating to exercise and weight according to the received 'truths' of contemporary health discourse. Young women, including those in our research, do not simply read and internalise uncritically the pedagogic messages of the media and formal education relating to body matters. There is no direct line of determination between media imagery and the actions that some take to 'lose weight' radically. Indeed, as we shall see, their actions are often motivated by a desire to subvert contemporary discourse while 'apparently' meeting its ideals in the process of regaining a degree of control over some aspects of their lives. Such actions, however, are often subsequently psychologised, pathologised and defined as pursuit of irrational 'unhealthy' ideals. The voices of the young women in our study exude agency and courage, not conformity or passivity, with their embodied actions speaking metaphorically of the rationality some required when dealing with the deeply problematic conditions of their lives (see Chapter 6).

Indeed, listening to their voices leads us to the view of social theorists, such as McCarthy and Dimitriadis (1999: 198), that the work of social and cultural reproduction has become inexorably complicated in recent years, not least by 'the multiple contemporary pressures of globalisation' and the new 'and unpredictable flows of people, money, technology, media images and ideologies spreading out across the globe in often highly disjunctive ways'. This has, as they say, important implications for education, 'as educational processes are at the very heart of social and economic reproduction', implying that schools cannot be studied as isolated and autonomous structures 'any more than one can simply assume *a priori* the imperatives of a bounded state' (*ibid.*). It follows that we are unlikely to understand the voices of young people unless we examine how popular culture plays an increasingly important part in their lives and is reflected in their understandings or readings of how and what they are taught in school, again mediated by culture and class. As McCarthy and Dimitriadis (*ibid.*: 199) argue, we now 'live at the nexus of multiple "power geometries" marked by unpredictable trans-national lines of connection between local and global forces'. In this context, the texts and tropes of popular culture circulate widely, 'coming to reflect a material and cultural hybridity that does not fit neatly into pre-existing modes of nationalistic thinking and planning'. Popular culture cannot, therefore, be looked at simply as 'an autonomous set of affectively invested texts that exert repressive power on young people' but is always inevitably mediated by class, cultures and embodied actions of individuals as they move across many sites, including families, communities and schools. This has implications not only for how we analyse, interpret and understand disordered eating and the embodied actions of young people in schools but for how we strategically address these issues.

If we accept this view we are obliged to reject those of critical pedagogues who argue that, as popular culture increasingly plays an important role in people's lives, it must be explored as a kind of 'alternative lived curriculum' which reproduces dominant cultural imperatives, 'assuming high levels of predictability from text to subject' (*ibid.*: 200). It also leads us to question those theorists of media literacy (e.g., Masterman, 1990) who stress that young people can be taught formally to resist some of the apparently deleterious effects of contemporary media culture,

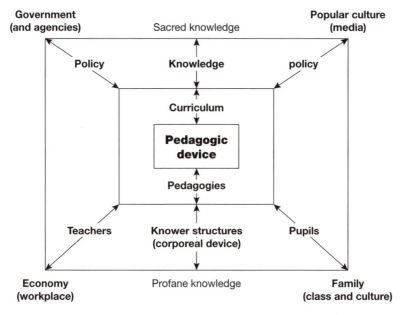

Sites of practice   Techniques of truth (obesity discourse)

Figure 1 Sites of practice, techniques of truth and the pedagogic device

such as the cult of slenderness around body imagery and weight. Both 'approaches assume that popular culture is a site of oppression for the young' obviating exploration of how 'different sites – for example, popular culture, educational policy, classroom practices – mutually inform each other in ways that help reproduce contingent state imperatives' (McCarthy and Dimitriadis, 1999: 200). We would add that they might serve not simply to reproduce but to challenge or interrupt such imperatives. The complexity of such relationships between various sites – and how complex 'technologies of truth', sets of discursive practices relating to the body and health, operate across them and impact upon young people's lives – is reflected in Figure 1.

As a heuristic device, Figure 1 facilitates analyses of the relationships outlined in the preceding narrative. It seeks to relate the variety of sites of social relation and practice in which discourses, health stories and particular 'technologies of truth' are generated and transmitted, for example by families, media, workplaces, official agencies, and their translation through formal legislated government Policies ('P') and informal school policies or strategies ('p') (see Chapter 6) *en route* to the curriculum and pedagogic practice, given shape and meaning by the pedagogic device. These relations and messages are recontextualised and 'read' through the embodied interactions of individuals and the mediation of the corporeal device. Tracing these interconnections may give us better purchase on how particular forms of knowledge – for example, from the biosciences and epidemiology within science and medicine – come to achieve elevated, 'sacred' status, deemed to offer perspectives on truth and reality that are more 'objective', detached, unequivocal, unambiguous, predictive and reliable than other forms whose 'truths' (e.g., about weight and health) can be made available to the many (or at least to any follower who seeks or heeds them), though access to the means of their generation/production, principles, methods and underlying codes is available only to the knowledgeable few. Some become privileged and endorsed through policy as official, educational/health knowledge(s) and enter into dynamic relationship with cultural understandings or knower structures, for example, around health and embodiment brought to schools by pupils and teachers from other sites of practice. How particular forms of knowledge and embodiment are privileged in the process while others are defined as irrelevant or 'profane' – equivocal, ambiguous, unreliable, contaminated by local subjectivities, ideologies and understandings – requires examination which takes us beyond 'conventional' readings of disordered eating in society and schools towards scrutiny of why and how the former achieves 'sacred' status (see Chapter 3) before infusing popular and formal educational cultures (see Chapter 5) and the embodied consciousness of young people in schools (Chapters 6, 7 and 8).

Beyond the cult of slenderness

Above all else the preceding analyses endorse the view that disordered eating involving severe weight loss and excessive exercise cannot simply be viewed as a 'benign rite of passage' (Steiner-Adair and Vorenburg, 1999: 107), faddish behaviours of irrational young people making the difficult transition from teenage to adult life. They have at least to be considered as rational actions of thinking individuals as they deal with complex, fast-changing, socio-cultural conditions experienced across many subcultural sites in and outside schools, not least the pressures for corporeal perfection and high-level academic performance. As these are pressures to which all children are subject, irrespective of gender, culture and class, it is no surprise that, although anorexia nervosa and bulimia are relatively rare in comparison to other affective disorders, 'the sub threshold components, for example, negative body image, fear of fat, feeling powerless and insecure, are prevalent enough among girls and women in many countries to be considered normative and an epidemic' (Levine and Piran, 1999: 321). Moreover, they are now extending to areas in which they were once thought to be culturally incompatible, such as China, India, Mexico and Brazil. As these authors point out, 'this horrible state of affairs, coupled with the astounding gender differences in eating disorder and the risk periods in early and late adolescence', does tend to highlight 'the need to think about what "eating problems" mean in the lives of young people, especially girls and women and, increasingly, of young men' (*ibid.*). Eating disorders are the third most common chronic illness among females in the USA: 'Research suggests that 1–2% of female adolescents develop anorexia nervosa, a slightly higher percentage develop bulimia nervosa, and the prevalence of eating disorder among preteens and younger adolescents is still on the rise'

(Goldman, 1996, quoted in *ibid.*: 107). In the UK the Eating Disorders Association estimates that over 1.1 million people are directly affected by eating disorders, with anorexia nervosa having one of the highest rates of mortality for any psychiatric condition, estimated to run at about 15–20% (see Beat, 2007: 1; BBC News, 2000: 1). Essentially the spread of Western ideals of a 'perfect' body shape through processes of acculturation appears to have rendered eating disorders unique among psychiatric disorders in the degree to which social and cultural factors influence their epidemiology, development and, perhaps, aetiology (*ibid.*: 2). As Gordon (2001: 11–12) notes, the one theme that seems to characterise the disparate geographic and cultural regions in which eating disorders are either evident or emerging

> is that they are either highly developed economies (such as Hong Kong and Singapore) or they are witnessing rapid market changes and their associated impact on the status of women. The impact of a global consumer culture, with powerful mandates for the cultivation of a certain type of body ideal, also appears to play a significant role. Equally important, however, are the contradictory pressures that emerge when women begin to have access on a mass level to education and a role in public life, and struggles about sexual equality come to the foreground. This may be especially problematic in societies in which the transition to a new female role is especially sudden and conflicts sharply with traditional forces that demand deference to one's family and submissiveness to men.

New patterns of food consumption and production and new styles of eating may also be factors in their spread, especially among young women.

In such views eating disorders are, in major part, products of the wrenching transformations of the twentieth century, including momentous superstructural changes in social and family life, social (especially gender role) relations and forms of human embodiment. 'Our' culture, so the argument goes, has been 'swept up in a web of peculiar and distorted beliefs about health, virtue, eating and appetite'. The pursuit of a lean, fat-free body has become a religion, especially among young women, although increasingly among men, too. In this sense, according to Seid (1994: 4): 'Anorexia Nervosa could be called the paradigm of our age for our creed encourages us all to adopt the behaviours and attitudes of the anorexic. The difference is one of degree not of kind.' In Rathner's (2001: 100) view 'it is not the image *per se* but the selling of the illusion of infinite technological or medical re-production of the human body' that constitutes an unattainable or illusory ideal. Calling on Shilling (1993) he reminds us that 'The more medicine and technology claim to control the body through its potential and literal construction, both fixing bodies and improving them, the less control people sense they have over their bodies' (Rathner, 2001: 101). However, viewing eating disorders simply as a Western, 'culture-bound syndrome' or 'ethnic disorder' (Gordon, 2000: 1) 'rooted in Western cultural values and conflict' (Prince, 1985: 300) has attendant problems clearly identified by Katzman and Lee (1997: 388). They highlight the cultural ethnocentrism in such thinking with reference to a range of studies in which 'self-starvation' is 'not driven by "fear of fatness" but the drive to instrumentally achieve self-determination when confronted with ambivalent cultural demands'. Indeed, it will become increasingly apparent as we progress through this book that we go some way to sharing their view that the image of eating disorders as a transitory, self-inflicted problem developed by young women lost in their world of fashion and calorie-restricting is 'a belittling stereotype' that may mask young women's real worries (*ibid.*: 389) and more complex concerns. As we shall see, eating disorders, whether mild or extreme, are not simply about food, nor about eating, nor, ironically, straightforwardly about body image or physique. These are often surface features of a deeper malaise, behaviours that many young women (and, increasingly, some young men) turn to when dealing with a wide range of contemporary experiences, not least of which are the problematic features of performative culture in society and schools. Indeed, our research will echo the view that, by emphasising slenderness, dominant imagery about eating concerns potentially 'misnames as much as it discounts real biases against women and their limited access to other forms of power or self-expression beyond corporeal power. Dissatisfaction with appearance often merely serves as "a stand in" for topics that are still invisible' (*ibid.*). Moreover, in our view, those relating to education and schooling in particular have yet to be foregrounded and explicated in full.

But even this language of critique is profoundly problematic and may lean excessively on the perception of eating disorders as individual recourse to achieving or regaining power and control. The danger in this view is that anorexia and other forms of disordered eating come to be viewed in terms of some psychological trait, usually defined as 'perfectionism' or the need to escape from psychological problems the individual cannot face or the 'desire' to regain control. While issues of power and control are central to understanding eating disorders, we recoil from any 'psychologisation' (Harwood, 2007) or 'individualisation' of such conditions (see Chapter 6 and 7). Such tendencies cannot adequately account for self-starvation and obfuscate and depoliticise the role that particular social institutions and policy strategies may play in the development of such disorders. Many previous studies have tended to explain eating disorders via accounts that either lean heavily on the 'traits' of 'the individual' or, at the other extreme, focus blame on cultural factors, such as the media and the 'cult of slenderness'. We, like Sobal and Maurer (1999), point out that reducing eating disorders to a 'pathological' condition of individuals diverts attention from the role that social institutions, such as schools, may play in shaping perceptions and actions related to weight (*fatness* and *thinness*). It also obstructs development of new frameworks within which to theorise research on eating disorders which move beyond notions of anorexia and other forms of disordered eating as *individual pathology* towards an understanding of disordered eating 'within its socio-cultural, political and gender-specific contexts' (Malson, 1998: xi).

The pedagogical implications of misrecognition

The 'causes' of eating disorders are multiple and complex and it is not the purpose of this book either to deal specifically with their aetiology or associated debates. We simply highlight that cultural over-evaluation of thinness and vilification of 'bodies' that fall outside a mesomorphic norm help set the stage for the high prevalence of body dissatisfaction and dieting. That these are precursors of disordered eating remains a central, powerful and enduring theme both in popular media and among policy-makers and schoolteachers. This influential but overly deterministic discursive tendency has had a powerful impact on the way in which eating disorders have been conceptualised in relation to education and schools. Essentially, formal education has been viewed largely as an ameliorative, 'corrective' intervention agency, a potential 'cure' for disorder rather than a set of processes which may themselves have problematic, damaging and 'disordering' effects on young people's lives. The former view has produced a range of policy and pedagogical practices, such as media literacy programmes in the USA and elsewhere that are designed to help students contest powerful cultural themes. Critically, so the argument runs, eating disorders need to be linked to the 'cult of slenderness' and what some in the USA see as its effect – 'weightism' – in society and schools. Young people need help to analyse the range of experiences that affect their lives, students need knowledge and skills through such programmes that challenge cultural messages, enabling them in turn to challenge prejudices around the stereotypes, self-loathing and exclusion of weightism. Steiner-Adair and Vorenburg (1999: 117) feel we need a pedagogy linked to other forms of 'diversity education', consciousness-raising and media literacy programmes reformulated around issues of social justice and inclusion if we are to help young people avoid the road to ill health and despair, slipping towards self-hatred, self-starvation and excessive exercise. Recent health and PE programmes in Australia and the USA reflect these emphases.

However, we again stress that to centre so squarely on media images as the primary site of influence in isolation from other sites of cultural reproduction that are important in the production of eating disorders, though relevant and potentially useful (see Chapter 9), may divert attention from more complex and immediately relevant conditions of educational practice that are inherent in the form, organisation and content of schooling. The voices reported in this book do not detract from the importance of considering that certain hegemonic body images (particularly the 'thin, taut, slender body') are powerful and influential global exports from the 'developed' Western world, although we shall also see that those same voices rage at and resent such imagery. Perhaps even more importantly, they foreground the need to consider how this imagery finds its way into the socio-cultural fabric of schools, as well as into other cultural terrain, and how a discourse of slenderness intersects with other educational discourses and becomes embedded in the pedagogical field. This is especially important if we take it as read that no right-minded pedagogue would wittingly *directly* purvey the notion that a near-emaciated body is corporeally how a young person ought to be. Yet, as we shall see, this is just what is sometimes expected and required of young people in some pedagogical subcultural fields, including some areas of sport and across other terrains (in playgrounds or at lunchtimes) in totally pedagogised schools. If we accept that most adults, including teachers, do not hold such views, we must consider by which mechanisms a discourse of slenderness is transmitted *indirectly*; whether, paradoxically, it is constructed unintentionally by its inverse, a discourse of 'obesity' driven paradigmatically by the interests of bioscience and recon-textualised through discourses of health, PE, sport and diet and other curricular elements in schools to provide the measure of performative ideals.

Reconstructing the field

Our criticism of the ways in which disordered eating has been treated in biologi-cal and some social science thinking derives from a mix of feminist analyses adopting poststructuralist and social-constructionist ideals (see Fallon *et al.*, 1994; MacSween, 1993) and other theorists of social reproduction (Bernstein 1990, 1996, 2000b; Shilling 2005, 2007) who provide purchase on the fine detail of social relations, lived experiences and embodied consciousness in schools and other sites of cultural practice. From a poststructural perspective (e.g., Hepworth, 1999), anorexia nervosa, like other disorders, has to be viewed as a social practice constructed via a range of discursive practices in anorexia, medicine and bio-science. Bio-medicine is seen to have constructed anorexia nervosa discursively. As with other discourses, diagnosis of, say, fat phobia, in a manner of other social practices, forms its own object (Foucault, 1972). However, Hepworth points out that even within this perspective, as in some of the more 'conventional' bio- and health science literature, there is sometimes a tendency to position females as passive subjects of hegemonic capitalist and patriarchal structures and ideals. There is too little concern with lived experience and embodied action (Shilling, 2007) or what we refer to as 'agency of the corporeal device'. Frost (2001: 29, quoting Featherstone, 1991: 171) exemplifies this, referring to the

> capitalist manufacture of bodily discontent [where] Western consumer capitalism needs women to feel their bodies are inadequate, so that they spend large amounts of money on products to alleviate this sense . . . Consumer culture latches on to the prevalent self preservationist conception of the body, which encourages the individual to adopt instrumental strategies to combat deterioration and decay . . . and combines it with the notion that the body is a vehicle of pleasure and self expression. Images of the body beautiful, openly sexual and associated with hedonism, leisure and display emphasise the importance of the look.

In this view potentially all women are rendered discontent with their bodies and many experience 'body hatred' states. Again, emphasis on body image, on 'slenderness' acting as a contemporary metaphor for desire and the management of female sexuality, is useful in stressing the importance of the image/media in the development of eating disorders (Treseder, 2007). But our research, like

Hepworth's (1999), points out that this view does not fully explicate the complex relationships either between culturally induced images and eating practices or between young women, men and other elements of their lives. As we shall see, young people read and critically reflect on the signs, select those that are meaningful, enjoy and recognise the achievable, while rejecting (or inverting), *if they can*, the patently unattainable, hurtful or bad. They vicariously ingest the nice bits of lifestyle, the broader imagery of ideally how they would like to be. They do not, though, all have 'equal opportunity' to reject or resist them, given the pressures inherent in the social relations of communities, families and schools. With Hepworth, then, we emphasise that 'multiple readings' of media images need to be interrogated if we are to begin to appreciate their significance, not only in the aetiology of disorders but, more broadly, in the aversions young people develop for certain aspects of schooling, including those designed to enhance involvement in physical activity and health.

Accepting this 'multiplicity of meanings' means acknowledging the role of human agency and warrants more detailed analysis of the corporeal device in decision-making. It moves away from positioning females and males as simply producing socially constructed representations of body image. It also means addressing power differentials between so-called experts in community and schools and the relationships between their 'expert' knowledge bases and participants' knowledge across many sites. In Hepworth's (1999: 126) terms local knowledge (Geertz, 1983) is a form of expert knowledge: 'individuals who participate in decision making are the experts on their experience and the reasons why change is necessary to improve health'. Yet, in school, clear lines tend to be drawn between official, 'sacred' health knowledge and everyday, profane popular health knowledge (see Figure 1) so that some young people feel that there is no space or opportunity for their knowledge and 'expertise' on health matters to be heard or acted upon. In Chapter 9 we point to the work of professionals who are attempting to address this by engaging with young people, giving them 'voice' in PE, health and sport contexts, as well as to those searching across disciplines to establish alternative understandings and conceptions of 'health'.

An alternative mindset: finding 'authority' in and through the body

Treating eating disorders and disordered eating more generally discursively through 'regularly occurring systems of language' requires us to understand them in relation to the social practices of epistemic communities by which they are defined, whether among psychiatrists, health scientists, doctors, feminists or school-subject teachers (see Chapter 3). It also requires a positive shift away from treating young women and men as deficit systems or as causes of psychopathology, from conceptualising eating disorders as individual problems towards understanding them as public issues enabling broader consideration of the breadth of cultural practices in education, employment, leisure, health and the family that structure and limit people's lives. It also means that we should avoid 'riveting our gaze on the femaleness of the problem' as, in doing so, 'we may be eclipsing the larger and more difficult questions. What is it about being female in today's society that predisposes women in particular to employ bodily idioms of distress?' (Hepworth, 1999: 3). Katzman (1997: 72), for example, suggests that by focusing on gender differences in general and media images in particular we may be missing more immediate 'critical cultural toxins', other than a drive for thinness, that may be impacting powerfully upon people's lives. We share Katzman's view that powerlessness may have been confused with femaleness, 'in effect interchanging gender difference with power differentials'. Notwithstanding the caveats earlier outlined, we take the view that power may be a more valuable heuristic for developing understanding not just of eating disorders but of the relations of women and men to aspects of education and schooling more generally. Indeed, we are reminded here of Garfinkel and Garner's (1982) comparative study of ballet students with those of a similar age studying at a professional-level music conservatory which, presumably, presented a comparably intense, competitive challenge to students at the ballet school but placed no emphasis on body shape. It was found that the conservatory students scored much lower on an 'Eating Attitudes' test than dance students and they were indistinguishable from a further comparison group of college students:

> Thus, the specific pressure for weight control, and not just performance demands and competition in general, is a critical factor in the development of anorexia nervosa. In other words, it is the combination of stringent require- ments for thinness with the highly competitive environment of the ballet school that significantly elevates the risk for the development of eating disorders.
>
> (Gordon, 2000: 125)

Given the heavy emphasis on achievement and performance in the contemporary culture of schools, this dynamic should be of considerable import to policy-makers and pedagogues, not least those promoting health education in PE, PEH and other areas of the curriculum. The resultant cocktail of high performance mixed with somewhat pathological body-centred perfection codes can, as we shall see, have deeply damaging consequences for students' identities, education and health, particularly among those who are emotionally vulnerable and at risk. We ask again what are the cultural toxins in education and other sites of cultural practice that may be at work in pressing young people towards corporeal disorder, if body image alone is not to blame? Are schools in the UK, the USA and elsewhere environments in which many of the new contradictory pressures and tensions confronting females and males converge? Gordon (*ibid.*: 110) contends:

> Intense academic pressures, a fluid and unstructured eating environment, the challenges of sexual relationships in an environment in which the possibility of sexual exploitation is increasingly a matter of concern, all contribute to a situation that can be overwhelming for those who are vulnerable.

The voices of those in this study strongly suggest that the complex interconnections between these aspects of schooling and other relationships and social practices within families, work and leisure need further interrogation if we are to help young people achieve levels of control, responsibility and autonomy that they require if they are to avoid drifting towards disordered eating and ill health. Organising our thinking about eating disorders as a problem of disconnection, transition and oppression, rather than dieting, weight and fat phobia, as Katzman (1997) has suggested, may be a small step in this direction.

Finally, we underline once again that this book is not about eating disorders *per se* but about how the lives of all young people are potentially affected by the health messages mediated through popular culture and the pedagogies of communities and schools. Our argument will run for as long as 'weight' or 'fat' defines analyses and dialogue between the clinician and patient, teacher and student, or coach and athlete, 'their concerns will be sorted along bodily dimensions while other concerns are potentially erased' (Katzman and Lee, 1997: 390). We trust that the pages of this book will make it abundantly clear that 'weight' is not a pathological 'disease' but a social construct, and terms like 'looking fat', particularly when used by girls and young women, may be shorthand for saying, 'I'm feeling undervalued, without control, alienated and deeply ****ed up' by the performative culture of society and school.

No one discourse or discipline will provide a complete framework for formulating future directions for the prevention of eating disorders/disordered eating or understanding the challenges facing young people generally in societies undergoing dramatic socio-cultural change. But, if nothing else, we hope that our analysis will help to highlight the complexity of an important contemporary issue and illustrate that questions of discourse, ethics, gender power, justice and social inclusion have to be not only at the forefront of but integrated in curriculum and policy analysis and development if, as policy-makers and pedagogues, we are to effect forms of education that are conducive to everyone's health.

3 Sacred knowledge, science and health policy

Obesity as instructional discourse

Fat orthodoxy

> They're always going on about obese kids at school . . . the government needs to stop stressing.[1]
>
> (Ruth, In)

In the UK and elsewhere our personal and public lives are increasingly framed and regulated by an incessant outpouring of health messages relating to obesity and measures to be taken to avoid it reflecting what some theorists have described as the *medicalisation* of our daily lives. The 'normal anxieties' we encounter in relation to food, relationships, exercise and work, among others, are reinterpreted as medical ones and 'problems that might previously have been thought of as existential – that is the problems of existence – now have a medical label attached' (Furedi, 2007: 1). Indeed, like Furedi, we would suggest that it is now very difficult to think of any kind of human experience that does not come with a health warning or some kind of medical explanation, creating a culture in which we are all seen as 'being potentially unwell' as 'the default state we live in today' (*ibid.*: 2). Arguably, being 'potentially ill is now so prevalent that we have reached a situation where illness has become a part of our identity, part of the human condition', so that 'illness is now as normal as health (and wellness), something we all have to work on as something to aspire to and achieve as if we don't buy into this discourse then we revert to "being ill"' (*ibid.*). Even worse, in our view, we risk being labelled aberrant, deviant or subversive for not wanting to achieve or engage with these inherently 'good things'. Echoes of an earlier age when juvenile courts reached into the private lives of youth and disguised basically punitive policies in a rhetoric of 'rehabilitation' (Platt, 1971) reverberate in today's obesity discourse, whose proponents, believing that 'youth' and their parents and carers need protection and correction from their inclinations to eat badly and exercise too little, endeavour to reach into every site of human activity. Their views draw upon theories offered by genetics, biology and epidemiology, much taken up by politicians (see Chapters 3 and 6) and like-minded educationalists, and have increasingly dominated political thinking since the mid-1970s and the way people think about themselves as embodied human beings. This has helped lay down the seeds of more pervasive and penetrating forms of control involving systems of social management and self-regulation driven by targets and numbers, the commodification of everything, including medical care, parenting and learning in and outside school. In this 'politicisation of health' (Furedi, 2007: 4) one focus of political activity, engendering policy after policy, has sought to deal with the impending obesity epidemic, requiring regulation of populations by informing them how they are to monitor both their own and others' 'bodies' through constant introspection and surveillance. As Furedi points out, in this culture and political climate, unless we are seen to be vigilant in keeping 'our body' (and those of others) in constant check, we are likely to be considered irresponsible citizens, letting us all down, at great cost to personal and public health.

The manner in which the politicisation of health has been invoked and framed in obesity discourse and associated health policy in the UK and elsewhere reflects wider socio-political tendencies towards the commodification of culture. 'Instructional narratives' within obesity discourse reduce 'health' essentially to an issue and indices of measurable *size and 'weight'*, given numerical value through a BMI score. We highlight problems associated with the use of BMI and the fault lines, ambiguities and contradictions in the narratives of its accompanying discourse. However, we neither concentrate overly on the veracity of obesity discourse claims nor pit one set of statistics against another, replacing one 'technology of truth' with another. Instead, our intention is to highlight its discursive elements in order to demonstrate how its narratives sanction behaviours which it considers exemplary (e.g., weighing children) and others which amount to sanctioning excessive exercise and weight loss, such as are ultimately deeply damaging to some young people's health. The question we invite is not 'What's wrong with obesity discourse?' but 'How did behaviour that is potentially so mortally dangerous come to be considered so morally, politically and educationally correct?' For example, in April 2007 Jim Flint, Minister of State for Schools and Fourteen–Nineteen Learners, and Caroline Flint, Minister of State for Public Health in the UK, wrote to headteachers of all primary schools in England to

> ask for your help for this year's National Child Measurement Programme (NCMP), which seeks to record the heights and weights of all Reception (age 4/5) and year 6 (age 11) pupils. The National Child Measurement Programme is a key component of our strategy to halt the growing problem of childhood obesity and help children lead healthier lives.
>
> (teachernet, 2007: 1)

A pilot exercise in 2005–6 had been less than successful as some parents and 'year 6 pupils, especially girls, refused to participate in the weighing and measuring on the day itself' (*ibid*.: 2). Ignoring their concerns and a sizeable critical academic literature (see below), the initiative was now to progress with greater vigour and more concerted action by headteachers co-opted, with personnel from primary care trusts (health workers who would do the measuring), to ensure that all parents and pupils would meet the requirement of the NCMP. Advocating methods of data collection admittedly a little more sensitive than those recorded by the young women at the beginning of this chapter as they reflected on their experiences of being weighed in secondary schools, the practices of weighing and measuring were now to become universal in England's primary schools. 'Weight' and 'height' were thus to be acknowledged by all teachers, pupils and parents as primary indices of the 'health' of young persons. 'Health' as a weight–height measurement was to become part of the vernacular, the grammar and syntax of the pedagogic device.

How did this reductive way of thinking about 'health' come to be defined and rationalised as official, 'sacred' knowledge, reliable, objective, uncontaminated by the profanities of commonsense thinking, regarded as an acceptable educational practice in schools? The moral dimensions of these issues are dealt with in subsequent chapters. Here, attention is given mainly to the instructional dimensions of policy and legislative provision that have formed their backdrop. However, we are ever mindful that separation of instructional and regulative discourses is entirely artificial and it is their intersection that comprises the body pedagogies that resonate in popular culture and schools.

Instructing the masses: there is nothing new

Tracing a detailed history of change in the way 'health' has been dealt with politically and educationally in the UK is beyond the scope of this analysis, though we do need to register some of the subtle shifts that have occurred in how it has been conceptualised in recent years. There is nothing new about politicians thinking that schools are important sites for dealing with health issues. PE, in particular, has long been associated officially with the development and maintenance of the health of schoolchildren in the UK, USA and elsewhere (see Kirk, 1992, 2004). In the UK, for example, well over sixty years ago the Board of Education published its *Syllabus of Physical Training for Schools* (BoE, 1933), a remarkable document, not only for the amount of detail it provided on the teaching of physical education (then called physical training) which was no doubt necessary for a teaching force then predominantly untrained to do so, but for the status it was accorded in the elementary school curriculum. 'The development of a good physique' and the provision of an 'efficient system of physical training' were seen as nothing less than a matter of 'national importance', 'vital to the welfare, even the survival of the race' (*ibid*.: 8). The echoes of war, general economic recession and widespread social deprivation, unsullied by very few of the supporting structures of a welfare state, had much to do with the board's emphasis on the production, promotion and maintenance of 'fitness for health'. Throughout the syllabus the social and medical functions of physical training loomed large. An efficient system could help compensate, if not correct, alleviate or act as a 'remedy for all [British economic and social] ills'. Such was their magnitude that the board acknowledged, in a manner not always so evident in more recent health reports, that physical training had its curative limits while still, somewhat optimistically, claiming that the syllabus could, 'if rightly and faithfully used, widely adopted and reasonably interpreted, yield an abundant harvest of recreation, improved physique and national health' (*ibid.*). Health, then, was considered a matter of national importance but essentially the preserve of PT teachers and sometimes, where local authorities could afford their provision, school nurses, known to many generations of children as 'nit nurses'.

While further change, well documented in the PE literature (Kirk, 1992, 2004) occurred in the intervening years, it was not until the 1980s that associations between politics, health and education started to become somewhat transformed, reflecting wider changes in attitudes and approaches to health. Since the middle of that decade 'health issues' have featured regularly within PE literature, first in the form of expressions of commitment to 'health-related fitness', later renamed 'health-related education' and thereafter increasingly in mainstream PE programmes in schools (see Fox, 1991; Penney and Harris, 2004). Indeed, in the UK, a commitment to certain elements of health education is now embedded in the National Curriculum for Physical Education (NCPE), to which all pupils between the ages of five and sixteen are entitled in England and Wales, and in non-statutory personal and social health education (PSHE). In Australia and New Zealand teachers and policy-makers seemed to embrace health issues even more warmly and explicitly, as is reflected in the subject nomenclature physical education *and* health (PEH) rather than simply PE. Moreover, many health discourses and practices now extend far beyond the boundaries of PE or PEH as subjects into a variety of school and community initiatives relating to exercise and food (see Chapter 5), all, in one way or another, expressing what we have elsewhere described as 'body perfection codes' (Evans and Davies, 2004: 207). These consist of principles that generate curricular and pedagogic modalities that variously focus on the body as: imperfect, whether through circumstances of one's social class or poverty, or through self-neglect; unfinished and to be ameliorated through physical therapy (for example, circuit training, fitness through sport, better diet); or threatened by the risks of modernity (or overeating and inactive lifestyles) and, therefore, in need of being supervised and changed (Evans *et al.*, 2004a).

Since the early 1980s such initiatives have been increasingly driven and legitimised by influences outside the educational establishment, embodied, for example, in World Health Organisation (WHO, 1998), British Heart Foundation (BHF, 1999), UK central government (House of Commons, 2001; National Audit Office, 2001), US Surgeon General (USDHHS, 1996, 2001) and Foresight (2005, 2007) reports. Drawing on data from a variety of sources, all have reported increasing health risks facing populations, not just those of Britain and the USA but globally. Couched in language of 'epidemic' and 'disease', report after report (e.g., Royal College of Physicians, 2004; Foresight, 2005, 2007) has warned of the dire state of Britain's health and, specifically, the rising tide of obesity, requiring action by central government, the food industry, the medical profession and schools to help the population take more exercise, eat properly and lose weight. So serious is this threat officially regarded in the UK that in 2004 the Secretary of State for Health, John Reid, announced a White Paper to tackle obesity (DoH, 2005b) and the Media and Culture Secretary, Tessa Jowell, hinted at a ban on junk-food advertising on children's television. Her department also claimed as a main cause for concern that 'many teachers believe that the government target of schools providing two hours of organized physical activity a week is impossible in the current curriculum' (*Guardian*, 2004: 1). Amid persistent and apparently irrefutable claims that obesity levels were continuing to rise, placing the majority of the population at serious health risk, Health Minister Caroline Flint was in 2006 appointed 'Minister for Fitness' with the task of getting people to boost activity levels to curb predicted rising levels of obesity. Subsequently, Foresight (2007), without any reference to the problems of either modelling or predicting population states (relating in this case to conditions of ill health) over forty years hence, confidently asserted:

> By 2050 60% of men and 40% of women could be clinically obese. Without action, obesity related diseases will cost an extra $45 billion per year requiring greater change than anything tried so far, and at multiple levels: personal, family, community and national [involving] partnerships between govern- ment, science, business and civil society.
>
> (Foresight, 2007: Summary, 2)

Thus 'health education' – or rather weight management programme interventions – are to achieve ubiquitous presence within totally pedagogised communities and totally pedagogised schools (see Chapter 6). More cautionary voices demonstrating that the available data did not support claims of an 'obesity epidemic', or that obesity can properly be termed an 'epidemic' or 'disease', were largely unheeded or dismissed as irrelevant (see Campos *et al.*, 2006; Gard and Wright, 2005).

Such notions have come to dominate the discursive terrain and now form part of the cultural fabric that defines our daily lives. Suitably armed with this *lingua franca*, political and media interests in education and health have effectively produced an environment in which 'crises' around 'standards' of health and edu- cation are readily constructed and to which government policy is the 'natural' response (see Warmington *et al.*, 2005). In one month, for example, the *Guardian* (one of Britain's 'heavyweight' daily newspapers) reported:

> 6 January: 'Traffic light' diet helps obese children slim
> 8 January: Obesity: rising fears of cancer time bomb
> 9 January: Pupils under seven to get free fruit
> 14 January: Jowell: no ban on junk food ads
> 18 January: Obese told: it's up to you
> 18 January: Celeb mag to tackle UK's health crisis
> 26 January: Coke logo banished from British schools
> 27 January: Pressure grows for curbs on junk food ads
> 30 January 2004: Fat test shows Manchester really is larger than life

Were we to look at the headlines of the more populist, tabloid newspapers in the UK, we would find an even more alarmist take on 'the crisis' putatively blighting our daily lives. For example, 'Campaign to tackle the perils of obesity . . . Weighty Britain . . . It's a national epidemic and we have to do something about it before it's too late' (*Daily Mirror*, 29/8/2006); 'Obesity is deadlier than smoking and can knock 13 years off your life' (*Daily Mail*, 17/10/2007); '14st Size 18 . . . Aged 9' (*Sun*, 28/2/2006); 'War on obesity: docs fight new black death' (*Daily Mirror*, 2004b). In the latter it was claimed that 'in 2002, 70% of men and 63% of women are either overweight or obese' and among the catalogue of risk factors, 'the terrifying increase in the number of children with Type 2 diabetes' and 'early death, heart disease, breast cancer, diabetes, colorectal cancer' (the list goes on) were paraded. The narrative was as proud with fact and certainty as it was loaded with emotion and intention to engender anxiety, fear and alarm.

These discursive tendencies are not peculiar to the UK. In Australia, for example, the Labor Party similarly announced plans for a healthier and more active lifestyle (Lundy and Gillard, 2003). Subsequently, its partisan press has relentlessly echoed that party's concern for the nation's health, for example: 'a SQUAD of anti-obesity health experts will knock on Sydney's doors in a grassroots effort to fight the childhood obesity epidemic' (*Daily Telegraph*, 2006: 1) while, from *HHS News* in the USA, we learned that 'Overweight and obesity threaten US health gains' (Thompson, 2001: 1). While perhaps not usually reaching the emotive depths of British tabloids, we could find close equivalents of the kind of reporting described above in other countries, too. Central government action, further restraint on the food industry, better diets and schools are invariably identified as 'key settings for public health strategies to prevent and decrease the prevalence of overweight and obesity' (USDHHS, 2001: 18) in the USA, UK and elsewhere. More policy to solve a crisis, more 'health education', more time for intensive physical activity and better school diets have become the shibboleths of the vast industry of health 'experts' operating in and outside the schools.

Allocating blame: good food, bad food – good citizens, bad citizens

Why are these discursive trends so worrying? Even a cursory reading of the aforementioned reports reveals that moral as well as medical overtones litter their pages (see Chapter 4) in the form of incantations about the 'right' amount of exercise, the 'right diet' and the 'correct' body shape. It is hardly surprising, then, that we find alongside obesity discourse a data set suggesting that levels of 'body disaffection' and eating disorders, such as anorexia nervosa and bulimia, especially among women and young girls, are higher than ever (Grogan, 1999; Treseder, 2007). Indeed, in the UK it is claimed that data on 'obesity' are revealing a new 'class divide' in relation to eating, telling the 'real story' of a divided nation. Reflecting the somewhat patronising and evaluative overtones that characterise this field, the diets of some children in 'the lower social classes' are 'scandalous', according to Professor Philip James, chairman of the London-based International Obesity Task Force and 'social divisions in health are getting worse' (*Sunday Times*, 2003: 14). In this view there has been a 'proletarianisation of fat' in which 'the overweight', once admired, are now despised. Whereas twenty years ago fat was a 'feminist issue', today we might argue that it is a class issue (*ibid*.; Campos, 2004). While it may or may not still be the case that 'it's the rich what get the pleasure, the poor what get the blame', it seems that the working classes get fatter from lack of exercise and poor diet while the middle classes get thin.

The simplicity of these arguments that caricature value systems around eating, fat and exercise is deeply disturbing and belies the complexity of the research evidence. It obscures not only the common 'desires' that 'the classes' may have to eat well, exercise and get healthy (Schools Heath Education Unit, 2003) but the way in which such opportunities to achieve these things are differently loaded by social location and wealth. In the USA the relationship between socio-economic status and overweight in girls is weaker than it is for women: girls from lower-income families have not consistently been found to be overweight compared to girls from higher-income families (USDHHS, 2001: 14). It is not that class differences are unimportant; on the contrary, data on weight, exercise and food are profoundly classed and cultured (Bourdieu, 1978) and should be located socially and culturally to be properly understood. But at the moment uncertain facts are traded as certainties, with strong evaluative overtones. Such discourse has helped nurture a variety of popular (e.g., celebrity chef) and policy (e.g., DoH, 2005a and b) interventions aimed at instructing pupils and their parents how and what they should eat in and outside schools, and it provides cultural resources to stigmatise and stereotype those who do not (or cannot) subscribe to recommended eating ideals. 'Getting fat' has class and cultural (especially gendered) implications, and its attendant discourse simultaneously positions as it labels those who cannot or will not take steps to avoid it within the social hierarchies of society and schools (see Chapter 6).

Given these cultural tendencies, it is not a good time to be either fat or poor in the UK or elsewhere in the Western world. Although the aetiology of obesity is described neutrally in the biomedical research and reports of the kind mentioned earlier as essentially a positive imbalance between energy ingested and energy expended, as a social practice it is regarded as neither innocently neutral nor value free (Cogan, 1999; Evans, 2003). Indeed Saukko (1999) argues that theories of obesity and anorexia, like many other theories of 'deviant' behaviour, tell us more about the norms of our times, which currently idealise individual independence and strength, than about eating. As Ritenbaugh (1982: 352) points out, the terms *obesity* and *overweight* have become 'the biomedical gloss for the moral failings of gluttony and sloth'. Individual control and fear of non-control are important themes in American society and obesity is a visual representation of non-control. Such socio-cultural tendencies are now equally evident in the UK and elsewhere (Evans *et al.*, 2002b; Gard and Wright, 2001). In the blame-the-victim culture that this nurtures fat is interpreted as an outward sign of neglect of one's corporeal self; a condition considered as shameful, dirty or irresponsibly ill, in effect, reproducing and institutionalising moral beliefs about the body and citizens. At the extreme, it exhorts people to develop embodied relationships based on fear, anxiety, guilt and regulation (Gordon, 2000, 2001) that underpin obesity panics, obsessive attention to 'self-control' through diet, exercise and even more extreme measures to achieve contemporary, slim ideals.

In the UK, then, we are purportedly getting simultaneously fatter and thinner; or rather, some (the working classes) are getting fat while others are getting thin. We are either eating too much or too little, exercising in excess or not enough. Moreover, more than two out of three people, at the latest count, are simply 'overweight', standing on the edge of the obesity abyss unless they eat the right food and take proper measures to exercise and get thin. The uncertainties generated by such shifting evidence and recommendations around exercise and food implicit in this discourse can be deeply unsettling and have a profound effect on the identities of children in schools where adults and young people can never achieve enough of the 'right knowledge' and certainty to guide what they ought to do in their own and others' interests. As we shall see, for the young people in our study, this had damaging psychological consequences as they attempted to live the experience of unattainable, corporeal ideals.

Reading the obesity literature: identifying its instructional tendencies and tropes

How might we read and interpret this literature where facts, ideology and assertion trade side by side as knowledge in the health fields (see Austin, 1999; Evans, 2003; Gard, 2004a and b; Gard and Wright, 2005) and identify its essential, instructional tropes? In the UK, the USA, Canada, Australia and elsewhere a subtle but significant shift has occurred in the *instructional* discourse that has underscored and legitimised developments in schools over the last two decades or so. This shift is reflected in the titles of the 1996 and 2001 Surgeon General reports in the USA and in similar texts in the UK. Whereas the USDHHS report *Physical Activity and Health* (1996) focused essentially on increasing levels of activity in the population in the USA, 2001's *Call to Action to Prevent and Decrease Overweight and Obesity* centred on 'weight' as the prime topic of concern. In the UK, prior to 2000, 'obesity' and weight issues barely received a mention by central government spokespeople, health advising agencies or professional PE texts. In the early 1990s, for example, important texts defining 'current issues' in PE (Armstrong and Sparkes, 1991; Armstrong, 1990, 1992) provided ample space for 'health issues' but reference to 'obesity' was largely incidental and there was explicit rejection of a narrow, instrumental or narcissistic focus on health in favour of programmes 'concerned with facilitating behaviours rather than the measurement of fitness' and more educationally informed notions of health promotion in schools (Fox, 1991: 124). These texts are a far cry from more recent endeavours in obesity literature and teacher professional discourse to rationalise the place and space for PE in schools in terms of its capacity not only to produce excellence in sport but to check the otherwise inexorable progress of obesity. For example, *Insight Media* (2007: 9) listed as its offerings on physical education on DVD: *The Weight Epidemic: Weighty Solutions*; *Childhood Obesity: Reversing the Trend*; *The Hows and Whys of Obesity*; *Obesity and the Relative Role of Exercise and Genetics*; and *Exercise as an Antidote for Obesity*. What began in the early 1980s and 1990s as concern for physical activity and exercise levels within more holistic conceptions of health is being reduced to a 'weight problem' and the business of measuring it, making people eat properly, get active and, ideally, become thin.

At one level this slippage in instructional discourse is unsurprising. Given the difficulties registered throughout the 1990s of measuring activity and defining levels at which it is beneficial to health, it is, perhaps, understandable that policy-makers and professionals with vested interests in PE and health should have turned their attention to what, on the surface, seemed 'auditable', 'objective' and reliable personal and national measures of individual or collective waistlines or body mass. What better indices of the efficacy of public policy on education and health in and outside schools than whether it has made people less heavy and manifestly more thin? This approach was reflected, at one level, in 2004 in the UK government's target 'to halt the increase in obesity among children under the age of 11 by 2010', which had grown from 9.6 per cent in 1995 to 13.7 per cent by 2003 (see National Audit Office, 2001, 2006). This target is jointly owned as a public service agreement by the Department of Health, the Department for Culture, Media and Sport and the Department for Education and Skills, while another requires Ofsted, England's school inspection service, to monitor from 2006 the weight and health of children in all primary schools.

These changes also had wider origins in the burgeoning culture of commodification that increasingly characterised schools in the 1980s and 1990s, reflecting the ideologies of neo-liberalism embodied in the measures introduced by successive Conservative and New Labour governments in the UK and widely echoed elsewhere. This culture celebrated accountability, assessment, target setting, performance measurement and league tables, providing 'objective' comparative data on and ostensibly facilitating judgements of schools and individuals within them. Obesity discourse and the BMI were given added impetus and importance within this dominant ideological frame, reflecting official desire for quantification and control. The deeper psychological effects of this culture and ideology are neatly summarised by Jenkins (2007: 18):

> To every activity is attached as a pecuniary value and thus a performance. To every performance is attached a target and to every target a league table. The targets may seem to be guided by what people say they want in focus groups, but in reality they are 'negotiated' by power blocs within the public service. Their enforcement depends on matrices of budgets, feedbacks and incentives, covered by quasi-contracts and internal pricing systems. Orwell's future, depicted as 'a boot stamping on a human face for ever' is now a computer mouse implanted in the brain.

Health was now to be conceptualised, configured, measured and assessed within this political culture. It was to be reduced to weight issues and their contingencies, levels of exercise and 'good' or 'bad' food. The BMI, as both a tool of measurement and regulation, played a central role in this process. With its assistance, in keeping with a wider political ideology of liberal individualism, a discourse of corporeal individualism is offered as 'the solution', where individuals, by knowing and avoiding relevant 'risk factors', are implicitly held personally responsible and accountable for the prevention of obesity and related health problems: too little exercise, poor diet, too much fast food. Schools, along with other key sites of social practice, including families, the media and the web, are positioned as pivotal in the process of correction, rehabilitation and repair.

Instructional fat facts

In considering the essential instructional tropes, key concepts and ideas of obesity discourse, it is important to remember three things. First, whereas fat can be considered, at least in part, to be a physical or visceral phenomenon, 'weight', 'overweight' and 'obesity' cannot. They are social arbitraries, measures constructed in the thinking of people such as researchers, doctors and risk assessors at insurance companies for whom indices of the body mass type were originally designed. Second, even when a threshold has been set for defining the point at which 'weight' becomes 'over-', it is another thing entirely to claim that it is a problem causally related to a person's health. The claim that 60–70 per cent of the population should now be considered 'overweight', a claim that is intended to set alarm bells ringing, is, in itself, of no more significance as a statement about a population's health than saying that its members, for much of the time, stand on two legs, unless it is considered in conjunction with a host of other data on exercise levels, diet and lifestyle factors, such as poverty and smoking. A weight-range norm is being pathologised and classified as a potentially life-threatening condition, despite convincing evidence that the 'ideal' weight for longevity is, indeed, 'overweight' (Campos *et al.*, 2006).

The third feature of this discourse which is of importance when assessing its instructional codes is that, although defining obesity is straightforward, measuring it is not. As others have noted, simply stated, 'obesity' refers to an excess of body *fat*, and it is to be distinguished from 'overweight', which refers to excess *weight* of some standard. But, as Brownell (1995: 386) emphasises, 'measuring weight is easy and inexpensive, while measuring body fat is not'. Consequently, 'overweight is often used as a proxy for obesity'. He also points out that the precise point at which scientists and health officials believe increasing weight threatens health ranges from 5 to 30 per cent above 'ideal weight', a considerable spread. Yet, despite such serious difficulties, differences of opinion and scientific uncertainties expressed in the primary health research field (see McGinnis and Foege (1993) for a US view of this issue), the 'health industry' – composed of health education experts, government agencies, many teachers, academics and accompanying voices in the popular media – has wholeheartedly embraced the highly questionable concept of ideal weight, 'the idea that weight associated with optimum health and longevity could be determined by height' (Seid, 1994: 7). Obesity is now typically defined as a BMI of 30 or higher (WHO, 1998). The BMI, however, is also acknowledged, at least by some, to be thoroughly imprecise. For example, it overestimates fatness in people who are muscular or athletic, does not register fat distribution and is an extremely poor measure for children and adolescents. Nevertheless, it is widely accepted and used in the medical profession and now advanced as a tool for use by teachers and Ofsted inspectors in schools. Professor Ian Macdonald (reported in the *Guardian*, 2002: 4), co-editor of the *International Journal of Obesity*, stated that the simplicity of the BMI makes it a godsend for researchers looking at trends, but he admitted that it is also something of a broad brush descriptor. 'Doctors like it and use it' simply because they may have neither the time nor the resources to apply more sophisticated measures that would provide more accurate and meaningful measurements of individuals' weight and health. The use of BMI and associated data on childhood obesity is even more alarming and unreflective. Researchers working in this field have acknowledged the difficulties of measuring children's weight, noting especially that 'comparison of data concerning obesity in children and adolescents around the world is difficult because of the lack of standardization of the classification of obesity and interpretation of indicators of overweight and obesity in these age groups' (Seidell, 2000: 26). Yet, the apparent increase in the prevalence of obesity among children and adolescents in many countries is still considered and presented by some as a particularly alarming 'fact' (Royal College of Physicians, 2004) and provides warrant for the claim that prevention of obesity 'should be amongst the highest priorities in public health' (Seidell, 2000: 28). The conditions this measurement tool discursively produces, *overweight* and *obesity*, combined with imputations of physically inactive lifestyles, are presented as a major, global health threat. Obesity becomes the most prevalent risk factor for chronic disease in most countries of the developed world and, as the product of global forces among established market economies, remains underpinned by conditions of increased wealth, sedentary lifestyles and altered eating habits. Wide variations in the prevalence of obesity and overweight both within and among countries which cast doubt on some of these core claims are noted (see the National Audit Office report, 2001) but hardly ever explained (see Gard, 2004a and b; Le Fanu, 1999; Stearns, 1999) and their other major fault lines are never entertained (Campos *et al.*, 2006).

Despite caveats, the official literature and its popular discourse variants set out to leave teachers, parents, health workers and pupils in little doubt that they are 'at risk'. It is claimed that data from almost all countries of the industrialised world and even those in the third world reveal a growing proportion of children and adults to be either overweight or obese and therefore, by definition, unhealthy. Bouchard (2000), for example, notes with alarm that about 50 per cent of adults in the United States and Canada and some of the Western European countries have a BMI of at least 25 (the threshold for 'overweight') and that the prevalence of frank obesity in childhood and adolescence has more than doubled since the 1960s, speculating that the worst-case scenario is that these latter increases will translate into even greater prevalence of adulthood obesity. Because there is no easy cure for this disease, prevention is seen to lie in targeting young children, adolescents and young adults through intervention programmes in schools and persuading the wider population to adopt a more physically active lifestyle associated with low-fat diets. What better rationale for the work of physical educators and other related health professionals, armed with skin callipers and BMI tables, could there be than to become the front-line saviours of fat humankind (Evans, 2003)?

Let us consider in some detail the House of Commons Public Accounts Select Committee Ninth Report (House of Commons, 2001: 1), *Tackling Obesity in England*. Having received views from a variety of 'expert sources', the report states emphatically and unequivocally:

> Most adults in England are overweight, and one in five – around 8 million in total – is obese. The prevalence of obesity is increasing world wide and, in England, has nearly trebled in the last 20 years. The most likely causes are an increasingly sedentary lifestyle combined with changes in eating patterns . . .
>
> Obesity is a major public health concern which is increasing throughout the world and for which there are no easy or short term solutions . . . [U]nless effective action is taken, over 20% of men and 25% of women could be obese by 2008, with important consequences for the NHS, the economy and the people involved.

Although the detailed National Audit Office (2001) report on which these statements are based is far more circumspect in its factual claims – for example, noting the problems of measuring and classifying obesity in adults and children and the difficulties associated with determining the aetiology of obesity, alluding to its complex demography in England, which suggests that there might be important socio-economic and ethnic differences in relationships between weight and being obese – these cautionary caveats are not reflected in the House of Commons report. But neither, for that matter, are they reflected explicitly in the *recommendations* of the Audit Office report, which also effectively reduces explanations of 'the obesity problem' essentially to a weight concern, the product of 'less active lifestyles and changes in eating patterns' (National Audit Office, 2001: 1). The data are rationalised to generate policy recommendations intended to influence the practices of health experts in local health authorities, government agencies and teachers concerned with personal, social, health and physical education in schools. A more recent variant of this literature, 'REPORT: Obesity Prevention: The Case for Action' (Kumanyika *et al.*, 2002: 1) further illustrates the discursive leanings of the obesity field. Published in the *International Journal of Obesity*, this article quickly gets into conventional stride. Without recourse to qualifying cautionary statements pointing either to uncertainty or ambiguity or cultural specificity of evidence available in the primary research field, we are told that 'overweight and obesity represent a rapidly growing "threat" to the health of populations and an increasing number of countries world wide'. Search as we might for the basis of this claim, it seems to rest on reference to other 'expert' opinion, rather than on primary research evidence.

This is not, of course, to suggest that there are no reliable facts and data in this discourse, or that rising levels of obesity and associated mortality rates are mere illusion. For some individuals and fractions of the population, in some countries, it may be a major concern. Our point here is simply that in this discourse, as in the House of Commons (2001) and Audit Office (2001) reports and in more recent media coverage of these issues (see Chapter 5), it is presented as axiomatic that weight (gain) is a (universal) problem, rather than either an expected element of normal growth and maturation or a product of near-global, contemporary improvement in diet and health. Weight, not health, dominates the discursive terrain via a language of threat, risk and uncertainty, individually, nationally and globally (Foresight, 2007). Our health and economic well-being are threatened by the spread of the obesity disease. In Kumanyika *et al.* (2002: 425), as is so often the case in this discourse, 'overweight' joins obesity (to swell numbers, we suspect) and exaggerate the problem espoused. Weight, especially the notion of putting it on, an otherwise neutral concept and quite useful practice in many cases and places, achieves the significance of a modern-day 'disease' and, by extension, verges on social and moral sin among those who fail to take appropriate steps to address it. Albeit unintentionally, even when there is welcome emphasis on a 'systems approach' to health (Foresight, 2007), potential is created for stigmatising those defined in the Audit Office (2001) report as most at risk to falling prey to 'the obesity disease' – for example, children of lower socio-economic and ethnic groups who become defined as pathologically unable to look after and alter their bodies by exercise and better diets and, therefore, stand in need of intervention, rescue and care.

Selecting for instruction: who is at risk and from what?

In epidemiological terms risk is a probabilistic rather than a deterministic concept, rendering inappropriate claims of either causality or certainty. But such caution is absent, for example, in the Kumanyika *et al.* (2002) article and the recommendations of the National Audit Office (2001). In the first page of the former, for example, we are led to believe, without any qualifying noises, that 'obesity is a major contributor to the global burden of disease and disability' and that 'overweight and obesity are important "risk factors" for a wide range of medical conditions' (Kumanyika *et al.*, 2002: 425), with boundaries between 'contributory' and 'causal' quietly disappearing. But what does this mean? What level of 'risk' is being discussed – the normal, the insignificant, the something to worry about slightly, the statistically significant, or the serious kind? We do not know; nor, it seems, do the authors. To make matters worse and the facts less certain, the article goes on to assert (*ibid.*: 426) that the 'risk of developing these conditions [of ill health] is greatest when the majority of excess fat is located around the abdomen [central obesity] rather than around the hips and thighs'. A similar point is made by the Audit Office (2001) report. Yet the tool for measuring obesity (the BMI) does not differentiate in this way and we do not know whether the tools used to measure obesity globally (as a basis for both the article and the NAO report) did so either; we cannot say whether the spread of global fatness is of the healthy or the unhealthy kind. One can only guess that a significant number of the people measured (for example, some women for whom the spread of fat is mostly around the hips and thighs) are 'overweight' but relatively healthy or, if not healthy, not at too much risk. Moreover, it is asserted that non-communicable diseases threaten to overwhelm care services world wide. Communicable maternal, prenatal and nutritional disorders (the traditional enemies) are expected to account for 10.3 million deaths a year in 2020, a decline from 17.2 million in 1990. Over the same period, deaths from non-communicable diseases are expected to rise from 28.1 million to 49.7 million a year, an increase of 77 per cent (Kumanyika *et al.*, 2002: 426). As everyone has to die of something, if communicable deaths go down, non-communicable deaths go up, with the latter rising starkly as people live longer as a result of steadily improving diets and health. Even to the ill-informed mind the figures suggest that if there were a dramatic decrease in communicable diseases, one would expect to find a statistically significant rise in the incidence of the non-communicable kind. And how are these expected figures calculated? We do not know how the forecasts were made because underlying methods and data are not presented. Even if they were modelling and forecasting of this kind over such time periods (over forty years in the case of the Foresight (2007) report) tends to be nearly worthless. And even if accurate, would they automatically signal increased cost to health services or merely changes in priorities and foci? There is simply not enough data there to draw conclusions of this kind. As for assertions of 'prevalence, trends, and economics' (Kumanyika *et al.*, 2002: 427), we can only take them for what they are – assertions – and no more. We are told that 'the prevalence of obesity is increasing world wide at an alarming rate' and that 'a clear relationship exists between average BMI and the prevalence of obesity in a population'. Of course 'a clear relationship' exists. Since obesity is defined as a given BMI value of 30, any shift of a distribution by increasing the mean will, unless there is a dramatic (and highly unlikely) decline in variance, lead to more of the distribution falling above the cut off at 30. There is certainly 'a clear relationship' but not of a causal kind. Unfortunately, the 'evidence' on 'childhood' (*ibid.*: 428) is even more alarming and alarmist and equally meaningless and shallow, given what we know of the vagaries of the maturation process and difficulties of measuring children's weight. We might respond to the statement that 'approximately 22 million children under 5 years old are "overweight" across the world' in one of two ways. First, we could ask, 'So what?', given that this is likely to signify a condition of 'health'. Second, we could enquire, 'Compared with what and when?', while noting that life expectancy has also increased in most of the countries mentioned, leaving us to ask, 'Do overweight and obesity therefore lead to prolonged quality of life and "health" or vice versa?'

How are teachers, pupils and young people, as well as parents, health workers, researchers and policy-makers, to read this data? How are they to deal with the ambiguities and uncertainties evident in this research field and the anxieties they may produce? Is it legitimate, for example, to read a normal increase in weight contingent upon improved diets as a startling trend and evidence of endemic disease? How are individuals to respond to the now barely heard but perfectly necessary notion for many of 'putting on weight'? Let us be clear: morbid obesity can be a serious health problem, especially in cultures that stigmatise it. We have no more wish to undermine the commitment of those who strive to address this condition than we would those who deal with eating disorders at the other extreme such as anorexia nervosa and bulimia nervosa. Certainly, it is to be acknowledged that, despite methodological problems in many individual studies, there is a body of evidence suggesting relationships between obesity and adverse health outcomes, including life expectancy (Jonas, 2002; Foresight, 2007) although, in respect of the latter, 'little or no increase in relative risk for premature mortality is observed until one reaches BMIs in the upper 30s or higher' (Campos *et al.*, 2006) and even then only when mediated by other complex conditions, among them levels of activity in a person's life. In short, neither overweight nor obesity can or should be reduced simply to a problem of 'weight concern', as occurs on the contemporary discursive terrain.[2] This has diminished not only our understanding of the location of the body and health in contemporary culture, particularly in relation to social class and the conditions of people's lives, but our thinking as to how health can be achieved by 'overweight' people without dieting and weight loss (Jonas, 2002; Campos *et al.*, 2006).

One of the dominant discursive features of the obesity literature, then, is how cautionary voices, ambiguities and uncertainties evident within the biomedical research knowledge base are unequivocally transformed and sanitised when used by state agencies, such as the World Health Organisation, House of Commons committees, health experts within academia and the media (Gard and Wright, 2001, 2005; Le Fanu, 1999; Campos *et al.*, 2006). Their morally loaded discourses become extremely difficult to challenge or contest, simply presenting as axiomatic that there is an epidemic of fatness afflicting the world. Given the way that overweight and obesity are defined, measured and conflated, half the population of the USA, Europe and the developing areas of the world is inevitably patholo-gised. These messages reverberate through policy initiatives and society, endorsed by a media industry, countless professional conferences (on obesity, food, diet and physical activity) and articles in professional and popular journals. The empirical question arises: how are these instructional messages recontextualised through the social relations and embodied actions of teachers and students, in and outside schools?

Constructing ill health and how to get well

Health beliefs, perceptions and definitions of illness are constructed, represented and reproduced through language that is culturally specific, ideologically laden and never value free. We fabricate and endorse beliefs about health and illness continually through the narratives of such texts and they have particular import as they enter the policies and practices of health experts and school pedagogies. Indeed, one has to note the form, function and content of such texts to appreciate their potential significance as a cultural toxin powerfully influencing not only policy and practice in education and health-promotion agencies but public psyche and the mindsets of teachers. First, these beliefs are presented as the voice of biomedical expertise. Experts have authority, power and authenticity and there are few uncertainties in the narrative, so it is nigh impossible for non-experts to challenge or contest its intent. Shielded from ambiguities and conflicts of opinion and evidence in the primary research field, readers, teachers, students and parents are asked to accept as a given that overweight and obese are inherently very bad things when, patently, they are not (Campos *et al.*, 2006). Second, both are typically conflated in order to increase the seriousness of the problem and to add impact to the central health theme that 'fat kills'. Rarely, if ever, is the reader invited to consider that weight gain is normal and to be expected or to question the veracity of such assertions as 'most adults in England are overweight', despite the imprecision of measurement techniques, the arbitrariness of thresholds used to draw 'normal weight lines' and the diversity of expert opinion in the field of primary research. Third, there is no invitation to ask at what particular point the condition overweight becomes damaging to one's health or how thresholds are established and measured. What are we to make of the residue of the population, those who fall below the threshold, who are presumably either normally healthy or more or less significantly underweight? Serving the interests of obesity discourse, these texts have next to nothing to say on this matter. Rarely do the risks of thinness or of being underweight receive media attention, despite numerous studies documenting that 'the relative risks associated with thinness' are far 'greater than those associated with even high levels BMI [more than] 35 of obesity' (Campos *et al.*, 2006).

This, then, is a narrative of certainty *and* negativity signalling obesity/weight, hence poor diets and lack of exercise, as a potential threat to personal, institutional, national and global health and economic well-being. Its instructional mantra is 'eat less, exercise more, lose weight', signifying a discourse of immediacy and proximity, presenting a here and now, on-the-doorstep 'disease'.[3] All could fall prey to its advances unless appropriate intervention, investment and action are taken at all appropriate levels, everywhere and all of the time. And by designating these issues as risky, this discourse has been instrumental in manufacturing a public health scare (Gard and Wright, 2001). Strategically, it creates a moral panic about a problem that requires intervention entailing surveillance and treatment of body shape, size and fatness. It instructs and informs how each and every one of us, the focus of the gaze, should properly behave. In the House of Commons (2001: 7) report, for example, it is recommended that

> practice nurses, dieticians and school nurses play a valuable role in identifying patients with *weight problems* [emphasis added] in providing advice and support on weight control, but practices vary. General practices should seek to engage a wider range of health professionals in this work, including those working in the community and school settings.

The upshot of this is that the social, cultural, psychological and economic complexities of obesity and health are reduced to the identification of a weight problem and its panacea – weight loss and eating 'proper' food. In the process, the health risks of underweight are almost entirely ignored, as are the body weight recommendations for optimum longevity that need to be considered in light of these risks (Campos *et al.*, 2006). The moral, evaluative and regulative overtones of such texts are barely disguised (see Chapter 4). A new set of value imperatives is brought into play. As Gard and Wright (2001: 546) have pointed out: 'the knowledge and practices associated with these discourses serve to classify individuals and populations as normal, or abnormal, as good or bad citizens, as at risk, therefore requiring the intervention of the state in the form of the medico health systems and education'. It is a discourse that allows not only health experts but teachers and pupils 'to construct those who are overweight as lazy and morally wanting, giving permission on a daily basis for intervention in people's lives (and at worst) ridicule and harassment and the right to publicly monitor the body shape of others'. These are extremely powerful and pervasive instructional messages defining competences and knowledges that 'have' to be acquired and embodied in the interest of achieving health – or, rather, avoiding ill health. However, even if presented with certainty through media, popular pedagogies and schools' body pedagogies they cannot and do not determine action without recontextualisation, filtering through the embodied experiences of teachers and students and the principles of the corporeal device. Indeed, we have spent time outlining the fault lines in this discourse because they provide spaces for individuals to interrupt, contest and reinterpret messages which are inherently unstable, given their contradictions and ambiguity.

Learning to be 'ill'

Notwithstanding such processes, it is to be acknowledged that these discourses are powerful, framing the thinking of young people in and outside schools. The young people in our study, like all others, routinely 'create and enact categories of significant difference, especially bodily difference, at home and in school' (Prout, 2000: 8, referring to the work of James, 1993), not in a socio-cultural vacuum but within frames of reference provided by obesity discourse. Hence, it is not surprising that categories of height, weight, shape, appearance, gender and performance become central to this process, or that they are 'employed to create "the child" as an "Othered category"' (*ibid.*). Within such a culture as James (1993, 2000) has found, 'stereotypes about what constitutes a normally developing body for a child assume great importance for both parents and children themselves', and 'deviations from these normative notions can create intense anxiety' (Prout, 2000: 8). Indeed, like James, we will later emphasise that

> the importance of bodily change for children can be found in their attitudes towards the altering shape and outline of their bodies [The way they come to perceive themselves, however, involves] far more than passive intoning of a received cultural stereotype. More complexly it is illustrative of how they understand, experience and use their changing bodies, and how, through

monitoring [both their own and others'] physiological body change, children
can be seen to be engaged in particular forms of body work.

(James, 2000: 30)

Again we emphasise that this does not always occur in environments of their own
making and rarely outside the gaze of 'others' who feel authorised by obesity
narratives to help them reconfigure their bodies, losing weight through exercise
and 'better diet' and, ideally, becoming thin.

Although young people do not passively absorb such messages but apprehend
and use them 'in experiencing not only their own body, but also its relationships
to other bodies' (Prout, 2000: 8), they cannot, especially in school, easily contest
or escape their influence and attendant pressures on their developing, sometimes
fragile, embodied selves to conform and achieve perfection. Such pressures are
intensely visceral because the sort of 'responsibility' invoked by the instructional
elements of obesity discourse signal not only that individuals should be responsible
but that they must look after themselves *for the sake of others*. Weight, shape and
size, so configured, are thus a social and a moral concern (see Chapter 4). The BMI
as a tool of both measurement and regulation, along with schools and other key
sites of social practice (families, TV, websites) positioned as pivotal in the process
of correction, rehabilitation and repair, play central roles in this process.

Finally, we stress that we have no wish to impugn the good intention, expertise
or core sentiment of those who report health problems, nor do we contest the view
that 'obesity' *in extremis* can be and often is a serious problem in some parts of
the world. Our quest is only to understand how and why it is that behaviours, such
as the pursuit of slenderness through excessive weight loss, potentially so mortally
dangerous, have become endorsed and credentialed as exemplary forms of
embodiment in society and schools. To this end we have sought only to highlight
the potential implications for the curricula, pedagogies and, more importantly, the
identities and well-being of children in schools of adopting an unthinking and
uncritical attitude towards the 'modern' discourse of ill health and its reductive
'instructional' tendencies shorn of hint of methodological limitations, ambiguities,
uncertainties and contradictions that reside in the primary research data bases that
inform them (Gard, 2004a and b). If nothing else, this acknowledges that problems
and questions we seek to solve through formal and informal means in schools and
other healthcare settings are inextricably tied to the way in which they are initially
constructed and defined. Has the culture of risk and fear being nurtured in society
by such reports and attendant policies and pedagogies created new 'hierarchies
of the body' that potentially damage the identities of children and young people
in society and schools? Has the cacophony of emotional reporting, ideological
assertion and political expediency that accompanies reports become a poor sub-
stitute for research evidence, informed opinion and common sense that should
define knowledge considered legitimate in the public domain? Is the current
uncritical allegiance to health education and obesity discourse that is intended to
help children and young people become active and healthy likely to leave them
feeling confident, competent, comfortable with and in control of their bodies,

or does it merely leave them 'corporeally damaged', feeling that they are to blame if they do not achieve these things? These, of course, are matters that require further investigation and all of them cannot be addressed in detail in this text. In the next chapter we turn to the regulative dimensions of obesity discourse to illustrate how these, when embedded in the instructional dimensions, form the body pedagogies of popular culture and the practices of schools.

Acknowledgement

We are extremely grateful to Terence C. Mills, Professor of Appled Statistics and Econometrics, Department of Economics, Loughborough University, for his advice and input to this chapter.

4 Fat ethics

Obesity as regulative discourse

It's my fault, my responsibility, me you have to blame

Self control of one's own weight might be described as a form of bioethics.

(Burry, 1999: 609)

Having outlined the instructional dimensions of obesity discourse in the previous chapter, our attention now turns to its regulative dimensions. Our focus builds on Burry's observation that the imperative to monitor one's weight has become an ethical matter. We explore the ethical dimensions of current health policy and practice, particularly regarding guidelines relating to weight issues, documenting how contemporary representations of obesity rely on medical 'facts' and create social meanings which influence how schoolchildren, their parents/guardians and family members are to be viewed and assessed as embodied subjects.

The variety of moralistic approaches to the body and health present in obesity discourse are rarely adduced for public scrutiny. Seldom in medical debates about obesity do we find discussion of the way in which morally loaded representations of the body affect individuals' sense of self and embodied identity. Building on previous critiques of obesity discourse (Gard and Wright, 2001; Campos, 2004), we endeavour to make this ethical context more explicit, the better to understand the positioning of particular moral principles and codes within discussions of 'biopedagogies' (Wright and Harwood, 2008) and body pedagogies.

We begin by exploring how 'thinness' has been cultivated as a universal value, leading to ethically dubious health policies towards obesity which can have a negative impact on the social identities and lives of people, as well as wider cultural understandings of health, weight and 'fat'. We then offer a wider assessment of the regulative functions of 'biopedagogies' in culture and begin to explore how regulative and instructional discourses shape specific body pedagogies in schools and out (see *ibid.*). In this context we consider how widespread concern about obesity enters cultural and pedagogical arenas as negotiation of value (Miah and Rich, 2008). In subsequent chapters we further illustrate how the regulative, when embedded in the instructional, forms the body pedagogies of popular culture and the informal and formal practices of schools. Health imperatives relating to 'eating well', exercising regularly and monitoring our bodies carry powerful moral as well as educational overtones. They specify what is deemed to be 'right' and 'good' by way of how individuals, parents/guardians and the population generally ought to behave. They are very difficult to resist or contest.

The ethical problems of thinness as a universal value

Our reading of obesity discourse runs counter to current, dominant, biomedical constructions of fatness and their associated solutions for tackling 'the obesity epidemic'. However, it should be noted that a range of opinion and conflicts of interest are latent within the medical sciences and professions and it should not be supposed that obesity discourse as currently fashioned is representative of all obesity research. Many and various voices compete for dominant definitions in this discursive field in which those of the medical and psychological professions are currently writ large, influencing and structuring mainstream discourse towards 'medicalizing weight and defining the clinical categories for obesity and eating disorders' (Sobal, 1995: 5), so that health tends to be constructed reductively as a matter of weight, size and shape, captured in the assertion that there is a correlation between being overweight and ill health and that losing weight will cure associated 'disease' (Campos, 2004). Emphasis on weight loss, rather than more holistic notions of health, circulates within contemporary education and social policy (Aphramor, 2005; Monaghan, 2005b). This not only makes no scientific sense in respect of the uncertainties residing in the primary research field (see Chapter 3) but may be ethically unsound. Many uncertainties, contradictions and ambiguities are often written out of, or remain unacknowledged in, obesity policy: for example, studies that reveal that being thin may have no more (and in certain circumstances fewer) health benefits than being 'overweight' and moderately active (see Gard and Wright, 2005). As Russell-Mayhew (2006: 254) suggests: 'The absence of obesity . . . does not guarantee health. Weight control is only one aspect of overall health and yet it seems to dominate health education and is clearly the focus of treatments aimed at obesity.' Indeed, Kassirer and Angell (1998) argue that sometimes the normalising focus in treatment of obesity has clearly been more on making people thin than on improving their health. While the purported risks of being overweight are constantly made public, we are seldom warned about the growing risks associated with weight loss. The universalistic demand is that everyone should participate in a culture of thinness on the premise that this is good for one's health. Aphramor (2005: 317) neatly summarises the consequences of this discursive lacuna:

> a continued focus on weight loss even on the basis of staggering failure rates alone is simply unethical. Perpetuating the 'size matters' messages fuels several unwholesome narratives: that everyone who is fat is unhealthy and would be healthier and better if they lost weight; that weight-loss behaviour is risk free; that sustained weight loss is always and equally achievable with suitable changes and commitment at an individual level; that it is primarily

the duty of the individual to fit and not an obligation for the more powerful in society to challenge narratives and address inequity, including size-based discrimination.

Not everyone has the physiological, social and cultural resources to achieve these things (thinness or ideal weight) and in some cases it may be impossible. Indeed, as Aphramor points out, treatment programmes that typically focus on weight loss have been found to be 95 per cent unsuccessful, reflecting this very point. The reductionist approach to weight loss as a calorie-in–energy-out equation may, as Gard and Wright (2005) note, be an unhelpful and misleading way of thinking about population levels of overweight and obesity, not least because it over-simplifies the way in which the body operates, ignoring that weight loss or weight gain may be effected by wider social, cultural and economic factors. In this sense, privileging weight loss may diminish patient care and, ultimately, the ethical legitimacy of current obesity discourse; 'messages may inadvertently have such a strong focus on weight and weight control that it overshadows health' (Russell-Mayhew, 2006: 256). In Aphramor's (2005: 315) view: 'Current weight-loss schema help to naturalise a fatness discourse that not only represents large people in offensively stereotyped ways but also fails to integrate people's lived experience as gendered, situated bodies in an inequitable world.' Within a discourse which assumes that individuals have equal access to social, political, financial and emotional resources, or is innocent of their relevance, weight loss is conceptualised essentially as an energy-in–energy-out equation. In this sense the 'obesity agenda succinctly epitomises the way in which biomedical understandings of health occlude social theory' (*ibid.*), excluding narratives which engage more critically with moral and ethical aspects of cultural ideals concerning the body and body politics.

Biopower and a corporeal ethic

In exploring the regulative features of obesity discourse we are interested in how widespread concerns about obesity enter cultural and pedagogical arenas as 'negotiations of value' (Miah and Rich, 2008) and how, in this process, instructional messages are deeply infused with a corporeal ethic, a socially regulative moral code. Obesity discourse prescribes particular practices that are presumed to be biomedical and value neutral but clearly imply concern that is both moral and ethical. Health is perceived reductively as strongly associated with body size and appearance, with thin or slender bodies being taken to represent not 'good health' but outward signs of self-control, virtue and good, responsible citizenship. The medicalisation of obesity has impacted on the way in which it is constructed not 'only as a health related risk, but as a social abnormality that must be eliminated and normalized' (Harjunen, 2003: 4). It has stretched the limits of medical governance by shifting focus from those who are clinically obese to target entire populations in the interests of preventing the spread of 'obesity disease'. Although now increasingly acknowledged as a particularly complex health issue (Bouchard,

2000; Flegal, 1999; Kassirer and Angell, 1998), obesity is reductively constructed as a problem essentially associated with individuals themselves, even if couched in a language of 'lifestyle'. Stripped of any class or cultural connotation or contingency, the latter is neatly sanitised, shifting responsibility from the politics of health to individuals' inherent 'ability' or capacity to act responsibly and change the way they live their lives. As Harjunen (2003: 3) observes: 'as a result of the dominance of medicine in obesity research, obesity has become strongly medicalized. In the medical context, obesity has been constructed as a physical and medical abnormality or disorder that requires medical attention.' Biomedical constructs endorse the idea that obesity is an individual 'condition' that needs remedying and to which the population is at risk. Thus, obesity discourse is grounded in an associated language of risk which not only suggests that intervention is needed and can be legitimately pursued by government or state agencies to regulate the body but imparts notions as to what is right and wrong, good or bad, normal or abnormal behaviour. In this discourse everyone, regardless of size, becomes implicated in the need to be vigilant against weight gain. It serves to pathologise those whose bodies fall outside of the norm by reducing bodily difference to matters of personal responsibility and lifestyle choice. To this extent, although the aetiology of obesity is described neutrally in biomedical research as an essentially positive imbalance between energy ingested and energy expended, as social practice it is neither innocently neutral nor value free (Cogan, 1999; Evans, 2003). These are bioethical issues wherein medical discourse on causality and treatment invokes a particular perspective on responsibility, the body and culture. A corporeal ethic is present which takes an inherently moral and ethical form in terms of regulating how we view the body and, in particular, the 'fat' body. Indeed, Saukko (1999) has argued that theories of obesity and anorexia, like many other theories of 'deviant' behaviour, tell us more about the norms of our times which currently idealise individual independence and strength than about eating. As Ritenbaugh (1982: 352) points out, the terms *obesity* and *overweight* have become 'the biomedical gloss for the moral failings of gluttony and sloth'. The fat body is a biomedical construction loaded with ideology and cultural belief about how we are to understand 'fatness' (see Gard and Wright, 2005). More specifically, in terms of bioethics, it encodes what properly constitutes care for the body in relation to weight and health. The use of a 'virtuous discourse' (Halse, 2007) and a 'rational ascetic' (Murphy, 1995: 109) are drawn upon in the construction of a distinct socially regulative moral code. Within a rational ascetic the aim is to subject the body to a systematic regime of 'rational conduct', working to 'discipline the body, to ensure that the body will behave (or move) in methodical and regular ways', predicated upon another inherently moral perspective that is seldom open for critique by emphasising the 'virtues of conscientiousness – virtues that are expressed in the careful and methodical way a person pursues a task, problem, issue or calling' (*ibid.*). This sort of approach to the body prohibits certain actions, such as idleness, and institutes methodical practices, in the case of obesity most strongly seen in imperatives for individuals to take responsibility for lifestyle choices.

Individual control and fear of non-control are important themes in Western societies where obesity has come to be read as a visual representation of the latter (Evans *et al.*, 2002b; Gard and Wright, 2001). A blame-the-victim culture reproducing and institutionalising moral beliefs about the body and citizens interprets fat as an outward sign of neglect of one's corporeal self, a condition considered shameful, dirty or irresponsibly ill. At the extreme, it engenders embodied relationships based on the fear, anxiety, guilt and regulation (Gordon, 2000, 2001) that underpin obesity panics and obsessive attention to 'self-control' through diet, exercise and even more extreme measures to achieve contemporary, slim ideals. These moral codes are spoken not only through popular culture but through the instructional discourse of medicine, carrying authority, power and authenticity, forming part of a process of health governance. In contemporary society, coercive means of manipulating populations using explicit force and oppressive rule of law have given way to more subtle and less directly coercive means of control involving a combination of mass surveillance and self-regulation (see Foucault, 1979, 1980; Wright and Harwood, 2008). Foucault (1979, 1980) refers to this as 'disciplinary power'. In his (Foucault, 1978) terms obesity discourse operates through a process of biopower which serves to

> bring into view a field of more or less rationalized attempts to intervene upon the vital characteristics of human existence. The vital characteristics of human beings, as living creatures who are born, mature, inhabit a body that can be trained and augmented and then sicken and die. And the vital characteristics of collectivities or populations are composed of such living beings.
>
> (Rabinow and Rose, 2006: 196–7)

Attempts to govern people's weight as a solution to the obesity epidemic take place via the normalisation and medicalisation of behaviours enabling the regulation of populations without actually 'engaging in coercive actions' (Gastaldo, 1997: 113). The provision of information about healthy lifestyles is integral to this process and draws upon strong moral imperatives that prescribe 'correct' choices concerning physical activity, body regulation, dietary habits and sedentary behaviour.

Pressure to obtain the right body size/shape is not, then, simply about being healthy but carries moral characterisations of the obese or overweight as lazy, self-indulgent and greedy (Gordon, 2000). In effect, feeling/being fat carries personal stigma (Goffman, 1963) which can evoke feelings of guilt, sadness and shame. The corollary of this is that control, virtue, goodness and 'pleasure' are to be found in slenderness and the processes of becoming (sometimes dangerously) thin, the sorts of virtues of conscientiousness related to making deliberate choices that are found in rational, ascetic conceptualisations of the body, health and medicine which accord superior status to the thin. Unsurprisingly, evidence is emerging that suggests these discourses have led to the marginalisation of obese people (e.g., Brink, 1994; Puhl and Brownell, 2001; Harjunen, 2003; Rich and Harjunen, 2004). Discrimination and stigmatisation occur not only on the basis of physical appearance but in relation to assumed moral weakness that is seen to be the cause of obese people's weight (Brink, 1994). Monaghan (2005b: 310) describes this as a complex process of 'moralising action, panic, fear and intense forms of social stigmatisation directed at bodies that putatively "fail" to "fit in"'. Such is the extent of the cultural stigmatisation of fat that discussion has ensued as to whether fatness might even be considered a disability (see Kirkland (2006) for a legal discussion of this). Garland-Thomson (2005: 1582) also suggests that fat might be a disability issue in two ways: 'Fat is sometimes a physical impairment, but it is always an appearance impairment. The fat body is disabled because it is discriminated against in two ways: first, fat bodies are subordinated by a built environment that excludes them; second, fat bodies are seen as unfortunate and contemptible.' While we would not take the position that fatness is a disability, these comments remind us of the covert and overt forms of weight-based discrimination that are articulated not only in popular culture but through official policy texts. For example, Aphramor (2006) has drawn attention to the use of imagery in health campaigns, including the World Cancer Fund, which displayed posters on buses in London with the tag line: 'Don't look like the back end of a bus, obesity can cause cancer: take control, find out how', accompanied by a figure of an overweight, faceless individual. Similarly, the British Dietetic Association suggested, 'Now is the time to deflate those spare tyres'. Once again, we would question whether any other 'medical' condition would be portrayed in such a fashion.

Obesity discourse, therefore, enters the cultural domain via a number of moral narratives supported by officialdom (Miah and Rich, 2008). For example, recent discussions in the popular press have suggested that a solution to the obesity problem would be to 'tax the fat'. In 2006, the British TV channel More 4 screened a Giles Coren documentary examining the cost of obesity to the British taxpayer, and asked whether central government should tax the fat. As Monaghan (2006b: 159) suggests, 'While discrepancies exist between official definitions of "excess" weight and everyday gendered understandings, fatness is being authoritatively and publicly discredited on a massive scale.' Moreover, in relation to education, O'Dea (2005) observes that obesity prevention efforts may result in further stigmatisation and discrimination against overweight and obese children and could reinforce the fat bias that exists in our culture. In this way, as Harjunen (2003: 2) suggests, the 'construction of obesity as abnormality and deviance leads into production and reproduction of obesity as a marginal and liminal space situated between normal and abnormal, health and disease etc'.

In this context weight loss is about more than simply aiming to achieve a 'slim figure'. Within this regulative discourse, individuals are deemed largely responsible for their own health and for 'making healthy choices', as if they were free of structural and cultural constraints that bear upon their opportunity to achieve the health behaviours prescribed. Moral responsibility is placed on individuals to have a good diet and to make certain 'lifestyle' choices regarding physical activity. By designating certain behaviours relating to food and exercise as 'good', 'bad' or 'risky', obesity discourse has been instrumental in manufacturing a public 'health scare' (see Evans, 2003; Gard and Wright, 2001). In the words of fourteen-year-old Lauren Hartley, who wanted plastic surgery, 'If you are not slim and perfect then you are considered not to be a real part of society' (*Sunday Times*, 2004: 16).

My body, your risk

Increasing emphasis on prevention of disease and risk expands the realm of health and medicine into the lives of not only the sick but, via processes of biopower, entire populations. The regulation of risk produces both 'population strategies' and 'individualising focuses' (Bunton, 1997: 229) and obesity discourse provides a particularly interesting example of how biopower brings them together as both individual responsibility and moral obligation to others (Edgley and Brissett, 1999; Wright and Harwood, 2008). Halse's (2007: 9) research on the use of BMI charts and biocitizens provides useful analysis of this process where 'personal responsibility for one's weight is constituted as both care for one's self *and* for others and therefore as a moral and ethical duty to wider society'. She suggests that within the contemporary culture of weightism one is expected to become the 'virtuous biocitizen' by ensuring that one's weight is within the prudential BMI 'norm'. She also highlights how new health discourses associated with the moral imperative to regulate one's weight assert an obligation towards oneself and a social responsibility towards others in a 'moral economy of virtue' (*ibid*.), categorising and differentiating good and bad citizens. The new, public-minded, socially responsible biocitizens are defined exclusively by how they manage the implications of their BMI. These pressures are intensely visceral because the sort of 'responsibility' invoked by the instructional elements of obesity discourse signal not only that individuals should be responsible for themselves but should look after themselves *for the sake of others*. Echoes of earlier 'child-saving crusades', albeit reconfigured around a language of intervention presaging individual responsibly to oneself, one's community and society, resonate throughout this discourse.

Moral codes and regulative pedagogy

Failure to conform to health advice or exhortations towards self-governance rarely result in official or legal sanctions; health is not enforced or achieved through totalising, didactic forms of power. Instead, governmentality is achieved via biopower (Wright and Harwood, 2008), invoking a powerful discourse of morality which regulates by inducing feelings of shame, guilt and anxiety (see Lupton, 1995; Rich and Evans, 2005). It is given expression in pedagogical form via body perfection codes that ascribe value and meaning to particular body types and behaviours embedded in educational practices focused on body matters, for example, physical education and health education (see Evans *et al.*, 2004a). Perfection codes determine what bodily acts are permitted and forbidden, the positive and negative values of different possible behaviours of and on the body. In contemporary health discourses such codes authorise teachers and other health professionals to foster certain predispositions and to maintain and impart specific knowledge categories, as Lydia (In), one of our respondents, illustrated:

> She [teacher] picked out this girl who was literally like this thick [pointing to a pole in the room] and she said, 'Now this looks like a girl who is the right weight.' That really upset me because I just thought I have to get [my weight] down quick, so, yeah, that probably had a big effect on me.

It will later become clear (see Chapters 6, 7, 9) that in a performative culture the correct size and shape become markers of distinction separating such young women from others as a measure of how disciplined and 'good' they have become. They feel their quality and value as 'good citizens' are defined through their relationships with food, diet and exercise. In the disciplined world of 'healthy eating' they learn that health, goodness and moral virtue lie not in 'what they eat' but, rather, in what and how much they 'can resist', demonstrated in how thin they are, or aspire to be. Young people such as these are pressed to make particular 'lifestyle' choices to address the 'risks' deemed to be ubiquitous. Health becomes primarily an individual obligation and responsibility (Lupton, 1999; Nettleton and Bunton, 1995), the message being that they are to take control of their health by making 'healthy choices', particularly in relation to diet:

> You just learn that some things are good for you and some things are bad and should be avoided. That's why I find it so hard here when they put a pasty in front of you, because I just think 'fat'. You don't learn that there are other things in 'bad' foods that are also good for you, like protein and carbohydrates.
> (Lauren, Fg)

Within perfection codes the regulation of the body is intimately bound up with moral imperatives relating to weight and, by defining whose and what bodies have status and value, 'body pedagogies' constituting acts of inclusion and exclusion carry particularly strong moral overtones in the notions of the body they prescribe and define. Individual responsibilities to accept correct diet and involvement in physical activity become moral as well as physical obligations. They constitute 'health imperatives' which impart a particular version of virtue and conscientiousness, accompanied by little to no debate as to whether, above and beyond biomedical health needs, this might be morally sound or 'healthy'. The young women in our study often alluded to the ways weight loss was not simply about achieving a healthy, slim body but about how individuals' characters come to be judged by others. For example, in Lydia's words once more: 'I had hassle when I was fat. You know, I wouldn't get asked out by boys. You know, every time I walked past a mirror I would hide myself' (In).

The normalising, regulative features of these body pedagogies induce young people to feel socially rewarded for following correct behaviour and their moral duty to 'shape the body':

In a way I felt like I started losing weight first cos there was this girl that I really didn't like and she was really fat and me and my best friends used to pick on her cos she was fat and we were really horrible to her . . . I really feel bad about it now . . . but we were really horrible to her and we used to call her 'fat' and everything and she started losing weight [. . .] I remember thinking, 'God she's gonna get thinner than me . . . and I have to be thinner than her so I can keep the power of being horrible to somebody' . . . and . . . I felt that it made me look . . . I'd got like a thing that having fat . . . like being fat made me look babyish and the one thing I wanted was to look older than everyone else and cos I thought I was, like, more mature than everyone else and everything and I wanted . . . I didn't want to look like babyish.

(Lara, In)

Clearly, these were not just incidental interactions but emotionally charged, visceral encounters, a form of affective bullying, a power play in which the authority to abuse another verbally or through social isolation was drawn from and legitimised by school policies and societal cultures which moralise and 'normalise' how the body should appear. These health imperatives differ from those typically found in wider consumer culture relating to slenderness and femininity, reaching and affecting a much broader population, including boys, as noted by one teacher at the centre:

Oh yes . . . particularly boys . . . I mean, we're not talking about people who are here who are overweight . . . grossly overweight . . . but other boys who've been here suffering from anorexia . . . severe anorexia . . . have . . . in their early teens . . . been overweight . . . and they've been teased for being overweight or . . . you know . . . they've felt sort of . . . conspicuous . . . . you know . . . being overweight . . . not hugely but a bit overweight . . . so they've done everything they can . . . including exercising to reduce their weight.

(Mrs Bailey, In)

In the disciplined world of 'healthy eating' they learn that health, goodness and moral virtue lie not in what they eat but in what and how much they can 'resist', demonstrated in how thin they are, or aspire to be:

I have only set out to eat [healthily] to lose weight, but I do feel that the messages sent out by schools, government and magazines have had a huge effect on me. When I started dieting, if I found out something was healthy, I had to have it. I felt that I was being different to most people eating chips and I suppose in a way that I would get recognised for being healthy. I don't know why this felt good, it's as if people would think I was doing good and in the early stages I did get praised for taking care of myself. If I'd go to the canteen and there was something healthy I'd have to have it, anything to help me feel better. The thought of something better for me going in me makes me think only good can come out of it. I am always feeling guilty, debating on what to eat, but for me the healthier options and messages if I was to always follow like before will kill me as I take them too far till I am out of control. If I see someone having something healthier than me I immediately feel guilty as I feel I am eating so much fat and it disgusts me and someone else is able to eat whatever and do whatever with their body.

(Ruth, Em)

Consciously and subconsciously, the message these young women routinely hear is that *they* are to *take control* of their academic well-being and health by making 'healthy choices', particularly in relation to diet, where schools were teaching them what was 'good' (i.e., fruit and vegetables) and 'bad' (i.e., fat). For these children, then, as for 'the obese', there is a perceived symbolic shaking of heads among the food and exercise 'experts' as their mortal decisions are ascribed to some flaw in *their* lifestyle. Given the social sanctions that go with this discourse, the bullying, stigma and labelling of which these girls talk, in association with being defined by their peers as 'fat', it is hardly surprising that many of them not only take drastic action to lose weight and become ill but become seriously depressed.

Conclusion

The above analyses begin to describe the way in which body pedagogies and their inherent instructional *and* regulative codes are reflected in the actions and perspectives of adults and young people. In subsequent chapters we will provide further evidence of this, while documenting how such codes have pervaded many aspects of the schooling and wider cultural experiences of the young women in our study. We will see that, for many of them, escaping the normalising effects of techniques of biopower associated with obesity seemed inconceivable. The pressures of being evaluated and evaluating and judging their own and others' bodies against unattainable social ideals were ever present in and out of school. Their voices highlight powerful ways in which the instructional and regulative principles inherent in health discourse relating to exercise, food, diet and body size are taken up within school cultures and can have powerful bearing on individuals' developing sense of well-being and self.

Focusing on regulative and instructional elements of pedagogy raises a number of questions about what properly constitutes care for the body in relation to weight and health issues and how medical-scientific approaches dominate public understandings of obesity, largely innocent of how their moralistic representations of the body affect young people's senses of self and embodied identity. Our data speak to the need to develop conceptual spaces that bring together and engage medical sociologists, health professionals and ethicists to formulate different modes of knowledge, constructs and critiques of obesity. In this chapter we have merely attempted to highlight the many complex and controversial ethical concerns that arise from the regulatory nature of obesity discourse in the hope that such discussion may offer more insight into its character and impact. We explore some of the theoretical and pedagogical challenges of achieving this in Chapter 9.

5 Popular pedagogies
Popular culture and media lifestyle advertising

Popular culture and the voice of popular pedagogy

> Advertising messages are acts of propaganda, challenging the faithless and the relapsed as they confirm the beliefs of the committed.
>
> (Fowles, 1996: 96)

It would be quite possible to saturate this chapter with examples of how various media, such as TV, magazines and film, have helped nurture moral panic by reporting the risks and dangers associated with obesity or, much more rarely, with being too thin. We have explored how the media relentlessly recontextualises health knowledge about weight and obesity either produced 'in house' as pseudo science or by scientists working in primary health research. We could document how magazine and newspaper articles spin 'stories' of the inadequacies of individuals or families who, purportedly, allow themselves or others to become unhealthily fat and potentially ill. As we write, in the UK, BBC Radio News, having 'contacted' some fifty consultant paediatricians, is leading with the headline, 'Infants being treated for obesity', claiming that 'Doctors say they are now seeing children as young as six months old in their obesity clinics'. Despite protestations from at least one of the paediatricians interviewed that 'obesity is a public health issue, not a child-protection issue', the commentary centred on whether such children should be taken away from parents and put into care, on the logic that 'In virtually all of the cases, it is down to overfeeding, according to the doctors surveyed . . . They are concerned that some parents are supersizing meal portions for very young children and have lost sight of what "normal" weight looks like' (Jones, 2007). Detail of methods, reliability, validity or nuance of data is never found in pseudo science of this kind.

Documenting how the media reduces and simplifies health knowledge, sanitising the ambiguities, contradictions and uncertainties inherent in the theories and findings in primary research fields, is an important element in any critique of obesity research. Later we allude to how such knowledge, when recycled, is reflected in the subjectivities of young people. But rather than embark on further analyses of the content of media messages and its reductive qualities, something that has been well undertaken by others (e.g., Gard and Wright, 2005; Campos,

2004), we want to ask a rather different set of questions. What is it about popular culture when mediated through various transmission modalities, such as TV, film, websites and magazines, that makes it so potentially damaging to some people's lives? What makes popular culture so popular, so potent as pedagogy, capable of reaching into and touching our cognition, emotion, desires and attitudes, the base elements of the corporeal device? The answer lies as much in its nature as a relay as in its content's seductive qualities, whether promising enhancement, amelioration, improvement or immediate gratification amid the otherwise humdrum routines of our lives. In centring attention on popular culture as pedagogy we can begin to assess how its form and content, its symbols, tropes and imagery conveyed through various media, take on instructional and regulative dimensions, as Ruth's comments reveal:

> I don't really know why I have such a fear of being fat, but I know that when I lost weight I was smaller and felt more daintier, as if I could then be protected more from anything, just a lot more safer. I think I really fear any comments of being fat as then I just feel inadequate and not as good. In all the magazines the celebrities and all the pretty girls are the women with the perfect slim bodies, anything else is slated by society. It wouldn't be if I was like proper obese, that would hurt, it's just being more than I'm happier with, that I don't feel slim enough, perfect enough and pretty enough. When I was dieting I got to a point where I felt smaller than a lot of people, and I felt sexy and I felt as if I was like as good as famous people. I had what they possessed the key to what I believed was happy lives as with the perfect body and the best looks life felt as if it could all just get better.
>
> (Ruth, Em)

Media matters

Lupton (1999) has argued that for many laypeople the mass media now constitutes one of *the* most important sources of information about health and medicine. As Lyons (2000: 350) comments: 'previously, medical practitioners dominated coverage of health and illness information, whereas today there are a variety of voices to be heard, including dissident doctors, alternative therapists, journalists, campaigners, academics and so on'. Indeed, one can identify a broader process of the medicalisation of health (see Miah and Rich, 2008). Certainly, the young people in our study accessed health information not just from traditional medical sources but from newspapers, magazines, television and other electronic media, with Ruth (In) reporting that she 'learnt about what healthy foods are from just what I was always hearing, good and bad foods', as well as 'magazines, diet articles everything that we're bombarded with on TV'. Growing research continues to highlight the importance of 'media representations of health and illness in shaping people's health beliefs and behaviours' (Giles, 2003: 318), critiquing many for their 'ability to mislead and misinform the public about health issues' (*ibid.*: 217).

We may illustrate the pedagogical elements of popular culture and their potential influence upon young people's lives by reference to Morgan Spurlock's *Super Size Me* (2004) and Jamie Oliver's 'celebrity chef' UK television series and accompanying books, which enjoyed enormous popularity during the period of this study, as did many other programmes dealing with food and 'weight' issues. Spurlock's documentary dealt explicitly with 'obesity' through an exploration of fast-food culture in America, with the narrator undertaking a thirty-day diet of only McDonald's food. Although shot on a shoestring budget by a previously unknown filmmaker, it went on to achieve global success. Jamie Oliver's TV career began with a modest production, *The Naked Chef* (1998–9), made for BBC2. Its success led to sequels to the book that accompanied the original series, *Return of the Naked Chef* (2000) and *Happy Days with the Naked Chef* (2001). *Jamie's Kitchen*, a documentary series, followed in 2002. In it, Oliver attempted to train a group of disadvantaged youth, who would, on completion of the course, be offered jobs at his new restaurant, *Fifteen*. Then came *Return to Jamie's Kitchen* in 2003 and *Jamie's Kitchen Australia* in 2006. Meanwhile, in *Jamie's School Dinners* (2005), a four-episode documentary series, Oliver took responsibility for running school meals in Kidbrooke School, London, for a year. One official website reported:

> Disgusted by the unhealthy fare being served to schoolchildren and a lack of healthy alternatives, he began a campaign to improve the standard of all Britain's school meals. Public awareness was raised and the UK government pledged to spend an extra £280 million on school dinners over three years, with Prime Minister Tony Blair acknowledging the policy to be a direct result of Oliver's campaign. Oliver was subsequently named Most Inspiring Political Figure of 2005 in Channel 4's Political Awards.
>
> (Solarnavigator, 2008)

While Spurlock sought to identify the source of obesity in the USA as overeating and fast food, Oliver determined to rectify it through better cooking, higher-quality food and direct action in schools. Both represented a new media genre in which the interests of popular culture and advertising collided to create a form of proselytising, popular pedagogy: good citizens take responsibility for their own and others' health behaviour. Such narratives traded relentlessly on contemporary food and health fashion, while appealing directly to individual aspirations and dreams. As one critic wrote of Oliver's later TV venture *Jamie at Home* (Channel 4, 2007), he had

> moved from campaigning about the real world to proselytising about the Arcadian one . . . from urban scooter bum with pubbable mates and the pancetta butties to a rural, wide-vowelled lord of the manor with a garter . . . it's less about how we eat and more about how we dream of eating. It's aspirational lifestyle soft porn: the wood burning oven, the walled kitchen garden. Mellors in the polytunnel, all organic and wholesome, and Edenish.

There is a suspicion that perhaps Jamie has cashed in the cred for rock-star rural.

(Gill, 2007: 15)

Super Size Me and Jamie Oliver's television series (*JOTVS*) are metonymic of the health discourses that were circulating widely in popular culture at the time of our study and formed a backcloth to these young women's lives, though they made explicit reference to neither of them. They did, however, draw routinely upon media storylines relating to health, diet and food to reflect on and sometimes rationalise their behaviour towards their bodies and health, though they neither simply consumed nor read them uncritically. Such 'storylines' did not 'cause' their eating disorders any more than, say, messages purveyed through formal education or in any of the other sites of cultural practice referred to in Figure 1 (p. 23). With others working in the field of disordered eating, we would again emphasise that although images, advertisements and other media messages can be counter-productive to good self-image and social acceptance of individuals' sizes and shapes, 'they are NOT the reason so many men and women develop an Eating Disorder' (http://www.something-fishy.org/cultural/themedia.php, 2005; original emphasis). Anorexia and bulimia, like other forms of disordered eating, are not straightforwardly about weight and food. They are complex disorders often with multiple antecedents reflecting many underlying issues that have led individuals to them (Lask, 2000). Moreover, the voices of the young people in our study do not lead us to be dismissive of media roles in the development of disordered relationships with the body and food. Although there are no unitary causations, it is, we suggest, at the intersection of media narratives of the body and those purveyed through formal education and other sites of social practice (in the family and among peers) that antecedents of disordered eating and, for some, more serious eating disorders are to be found. Our thesis here is that media messages do not stand alone but enter into a number of 'inter-textual relationships' (Fowles, 1996: 90), including with those purveyed through formal education, which may be particularly virulent. Even then, they are not uncritically imbibed, for, as readers and 'consumers' of popular culture, young people are adept, social creatures (*ibid.*: 161). Their interactions with the media are always acts of communication entailing interpretation, evaluation and recontextualisation in which there is inevitably adaptation, resistance, rejection or accommodation of the messages received. They mediate and are often deeply critical of media messages and their cultural tropes. The space for recontextualisation and critical reflection arises in much the same manner as Fowles (*ibid.*: 159) pointed out that advertising

cannot create social actualities out of whole cloth, and it is folly to think that it could. To believe that it can impose stereotypes of its own making upon the public is to hold demeaning and, in the end, unsupportable views about the nature of the public. Consumers do not all accept the idealizations in advertising then pattern them determinedly upon them, or there would be much more uniformity in taste and appearance than there is [. . .] Only when one re-considers the imagery that actually lies at the surface of advertisement can we begin to understand the relationship between advertising messages, consumers and the creation or mirroring of reality. [W]hat is seen on the surface are renderings of people in the prime of life, stripped of occupational roles, stripped of class locations, stripped of ethnicity, stripped of age considerations, and constituted as paragons of their genders. Missing is most of human life-work, duty routines, small kindnesses as well as unpleasantries. [. . .] Advertising distils from the variety of human appearances the few that will be accepted as apotheoses and returns them in perfected form to an audience desiring to see such singular renditions.

We need to address the parallel dimensions of popular culture if we are to understand it as a form of pedagogy and fully appreciate its potential impact on young people's lives. This means interrogating not only its regulative and instructional components, the messages it relays, but the nature of the relay itself.

Popular pedagogy as lifestyle advertising

We use the term *popular culture*, following Fowles (1996: 11), to refer to 'entertainment that is produced by the culture industries, composed of symbolic content, mediated widely, and consumed with pleasure'. Advertising transmitted through TV, film, radio, magazines and websites may be considered a subset of popular culture, intent on getting consumers to do that which they otherwise might not. 'Typically advertising draws on popular culture's repository of symbolic material (images or text or music) in an attempt to fabricate new symbols with enlivened meanings' (*ibid.*: 9). The creators of popular culture 'fabricate their offerings with no other goal than that it be found diverting and attractive to the public' (*ibid.*: 13); advertising 'aims at changing behaviour whereas the function of popular culture is not one of change but of maintenance' (*ibid.*: 12). Advertising has ulterior motives whereas popular culture, as in box-office films or prime-time TV, is 'usually designed for little more than immediate and pleasurable gratification . . . Together they dominate today's environment of symbols overriding more traditional forms of expression' (*ibid.*: xiii).

However, these distinctions have become increasingly blurred in recent years as popular culture, especially TV and film, has sought not only to 'entertain' and ensure that mass communication occurs through imagery that is both populist and inherently pleasurable but to 'educate' and bring about certain lifestyle changes, either in the pursuit of altruistic interests (such as promoting better health) or in market behaviour that favours advertisers' wares (such as particular foodstuffs or clothing). At one level the *JOTVS* may be considered a form of popular culture and at another they bear features indistinguishable from the 'compound advertising' which Fowles (*ibid.*: 11) claims 'occurs when consumers are encouraged to transfer the positive associations of the non commodity material onto the commodity', so that, for example, independence, freedom and friendship equal a Jamie Oliver Sainsbury's dinner. Oliver's books further endorse such connective ideals, claiming that 'food is friends', detailing 'a curry with your mates' and providing 'a menu to impress': 'if you've got your eyes on that special someone then this is the menu to cook for them. Not only will it make them sit up and take notice of your amazing cooking skills, but it's guaranteed to succeed in making them notice you too' (Oliver, 2003: 14). Jamie Oliver's popularity has rested not just on the quality of the food he has produced (which, we suspect, most young people could not recollect and would not want to reproduce even if they could) but with the lifestyle and culture he represents and endorses: the scooter; the spiral staircase; the basketball net in the hall; the vibrant friends; and, critically, the fun, freedom, independence and wealth he enjoys. In effect, young people have been invited vicariously to ingest nice bits of his lifestyle and the broader imagery of ideally how they could and perhaps *should* be, if only they ate the 'right' foods, became independent, active and thin. Food in this context is not just about or even remotely for eating; it is for distinction and style. As Fowles (1996: 17) has pointed out, both popular culture and advertising are products of the culture industries, 'giant capitalist bastions whose activities are governed absolutely by the search for profit'. Yet both must also be understood as

> artistic products, at least in their pretensions. The more artistic they are, the more successful they are likely to be. Only when the individual viewer experiences the communication as artistic, where symbols artfully reach through cognition to the layers of feelings and do so in an ultimately pleasurable way, is that individual likely to be touched significantly by the content. To make their content as delectable as possible, both advertising and popular culture pay great attention to style.
>
> (*Ibid.*)

To understand the popularity of popular culture in people's lives it has to be acknowledged that it is 'always contrived as if it is to be received by individuals not masses; to insist that it is received by audiences is to perpetuate its denigration and miscomprehension' (*ibid.*: 104). The potency of popular culture derives not from its ubiquity but from its capacity to seem to speak directly to individuals' interests, their personal and private aspirations, as well as their troubles and needs. In the words of one of our young respondents: 'Yeah, but people actually do listen ... I always thought like ... they were always aiming at me when there was stuff in the magazines' (Vicky, Fg). Even though such messages are interpreted individually, they are not received or read in a social vacuum but recontextualised amid the prevailing interests of peer-group cultures, family members and school personnel. As a parent, Mrs Johnson (In), commented:

> and they soon get in a group that get together and go on about diets and that and again ... it's like I say in a lot of like the ... cos I've found with, you know, like *Closer* and *Heat* ... you know all those magazines [. . .] Yeah, cos like I said ... they kept going on about diets and losing weight it made ... I think it made Olivia think that way [. . .] And I think if you're hearing that every day it's gonna sort of like brainwash you eventually.

But by far the most potent element of popular pedagogy is its commitment to the pleasure principle. As Fowles (1996: 105) points out, 'pleasure is the most important attribute of the reception of popular culture; no consideration should be allowed to conceal or colour this fundamental fact'. Certainly, at least in the initial stages of the development of their disordered relationships with food, some of the young people in our study took pleasure not only from pursuing and matching themselves against media corporeal ideals but from the recognition, status and distinction to be gained from being seen to be following popular representations of 'healthy' ones routinely observed and learned about in magazines and TV concerning eating the right foods and being the correct size. Moreover, as the expectations of popular culture become firmly ensconced in the informal ones of schools, they constantly monitored and competed against each other in the quest to be seen to be meeting the highest ideals:

> Oh yeah . . . lots of people at school will call you fat and everyone like . . . your friends analyse everyone about who's got the biggest thighs . . . who's the prettiest and stuff . . . You have to have the right clothes and be thin and pretty and everyone compares each other . . . everyone, like, looks . . . looks to see if you've lost or gained weight . . . Like if you wear a skirt everyone looks to see if you've lost or gained weight . . . and once the girls . . . the girls in my class even asked the boys to compare them all . . . like to compare all the girls and say who had the best body and stuff.
>
> (Tracey, In)

For some, achieving recognition and distinction involved taking the imperatives of popular culture to the extreme:

> *Laura*:   There were quite a lot of people at the school who didn't eat properly anyway.
> *RA*:   Oh right . . . was that through eating disorders do you think or . . . ?
> *Laura*:   Partly . . . erm . . . and partly just like not wanting to be seen eating . . . like teenage girls don't always want to be seen by other people to be eating unhealthy foods cos then everyone will think they're really fat and things just from eating that.
>
> (Laura, In)

And Ruth remarked:

> I take a lot of notice into the healthy eating of my friends (now more than ever), and if I feel they are eating more healthier than me it will really get at me as it's unfair they can get away with it [. . .] Anyway, with my mate, even though I knew she was healthily eating, her healthy eating wasn't the same for me. I considered mine different as I thought she could eat whatever and get away with it, but I had to work harder which meant eating more 'healthier',

which in my case was less fat, less calories, less food, and more exercise to just get me that one step ahead.

(Ruth, Em)

But perhaps the most important point here is that it appears impossible for these young people to position themselves outside of the logic of popular culture, to think of themselves as 'unmediated', to locate a contemporary space which discursively is 'free' from the proselytising, pedagogical narratives of body shape, exercise and food. Some appealed to and romanticised a lost golden age of their parents' generation; a time before obsession with calories, exercise and diet, a time when it was possible to take pleasure from 'just' eating food:

Rebekah: Yeah . . . cos when you think about it . . . it really annoys me actually cos like years ago when your parents were at school and stuff . . . there was not all the . . . you know people just had their dinner and that was it . . . there's so much emphasis now I think . . . it can cause a lot of problems.

RA: Yeah . . . was there much at school then about healthy eating?

Rebekah: Yeah there were posters everywhere and . . . you know . . . it's just ridiculous . . . and even with the young . . . cos I was quite a fussy eater anyway . . . so I think it just makes it worse . . . definitely . . . yeah.

(In)

In articulating such processes we want to explore further the role that cinematic imagery, such as that of *Super Size Me*, plays as a pedagogical relay, bringing particular discourses about obesity into existence.

Film as pedagogical relay: *Super Size Me*

Super Size Me was clearly an attempt to offer both scientific and moralistic commentary on the relationship between fast-food culture and obesity within the USA, and Spurlock not only narrates the film but documents the process of putting himself through a diet of eating nothing but items found on the McDonald's menu, water included, three times a day for thirty days. He always 'supersized' his meal when 'invited' to do so at the sales counter. Furthermore, because the average American walks only half a mile a day, he walked fewer than 5,000 steps each day.

Like other documentaries, the film draws on a variety of 'expertise' throughout:

Here's a documentary which needs absolutely no introduction. Why is America so fat? This is the question that Morgan Spurlock wanted to answer. He set out to interview experts in 20 US cities, including Houston – 'The Fattest City' in America – whilst at the same time conducting his own personal experiment . . . To eat nothing but McDonald's for 30 Days.

(*Super Size Me*, official DVD summary)

In his 'experiment' Spurlock enlisted a doctor, dietician, cardiologist and gastroen-terologist to monitor his health. The film's exposition includes the views of a number of individuals presented as leading academic writers, 'experts' on the obesity debate, along with 'scientific evidence' supporting a medical perspective on food, weight and health, as well as laypeople who relate their attitudes towards and experiences of fast food. Analogous techniques are evident in *JOTVS*, but Oliver himself assumes the role of both 'expert' cook and (implicitly) nutritionist, and the audience is invited to take on trust his view of food and health. Just as in the Spurlock film Oliver's messages are embodied in his actions and lifestyle, and his appearance is central to how the message is received. There is not space here to give a detailed analysis of either *JOTVS* or *Super Size Me*. Instead, we examine how both recontextualise heath discourses into a popular media format. How were meanings around obesity and health framed within and by these particular texts and how does this connect with our wider interest concerning body pedagogy?

Scientific and documentary search for 'truth'

Like other popular health media, *Super Size Me* resonates as 'discursive truth'. Nowhere in the film is it suggested that the relationship between obesity and health or how obesity is constructed is problematic. It is simply taken as a given that 'obesity' *is* a problem of epidemic proportions. At the start of *Super Size Me*, Spurlock announces: 'Nearly 100 million Americans are overweight or obese – nearly 60% of all US adults. Since 1980 the total number of overweight and obese Americans has doubled, with twice as many overweight children and three times as many overweight adolescents.' Nowhere are these figures challenged or explained, and no mention is made of the complexity of measuring obesity. 'Overweight' and 'obese' are conflated as potential health problems despite growing evidence that they patently are not. The subjects in the film are 'framed within a story that provides coherence to the evidence presented' (Hodgetts and Chamberlain, 1999: 321) around the seemingly simple relationship between being overweight and health. In various scenes Spurlock visits a registered dietician at a 'wellness centre' to help track his progress. During the first consultation the dietician measures his height and weight and comments: 'For your height, this is a healthy weight, I can tell you that. Your BMI, which is Body Mass Index, is in the normal limits, which means you're not obese, you're actually at the correct weight.' BMI, as we saw in Chapter 3, defines 'obese' as 30 kg/m^2 or higher, above the stated ideals of 'healthy weight', which lie between 18.5 and 24.9 (WHO, 1998). As we pointed out, it is a problematic tool for making claims about health, yet it has become the standard for determining population levels of obesity. In the film, analysis of the relationship between health and weight ends with the voice of the 'dietician' speaking with conviction and certainty of the dangers of over-weight. BMI charts are now often found accompanying media reports on obesity as a reliable measurement for readers to assess their weight status, as is the case with *Super Size Me*, where the expert voice drawn upon in the cinematic moment refers to thresholds of weight and height with clear, distinguishable effects on health. These become pedagogical tools for the public to make sense of their own health. In this discourse health is a matter of cause and effect, a product rather than an evolving process or state of always becoming. *Super Size Me* simply asserts the idea that being overweight and obesity are both pathological conditions, despite evidence which suggests that for many people there may be little or no relation between weight and health.[1] Little is heard about the complex relationships between physical activity, health and weight: health is simply reduced to an energy-in–energy-out equation, with excess of the former resulting in weight gain. There is no effort to draw on studies which have revealed that a moderately active fat person is likely to be far healthier than someone who is thin but sedentary (Campos, 2004).

Indeed, there is, in effect, little or no 'debate' on obesity at all (Monaghan, 2005b); it is simply assumed and unequivocally stated that here is a problem of epidemic proportions, whose causes and effects, together with 'solutions', require elucidation. *Super Size Me* adopts a similar narrative, failing to explore the growing research which has alluded to the paucity of reliable knowledge in relation to obesity discourse (e.g., Atrens, 2000; Bouchard and Blair, 1999; Flegal, 1999; Gard and Wright, 2001). Nowhere is it countenanced that losing weight might be dangerous to health, or that there may be many good reasons why people eat and enjoy 'fast food'. In this and other media, uncertain knowledge generated in the primary fields of bio/health sciences on obesity is typically recycled as discursive 'truths' within the media and 'educational' practices of schools.

Fat fear and its educational effects

It is hardly surprising, then, that 'fat', having been so relentlessly demonised in popular pedagogy, featured repeatedly in the narratives of the young people in our study:

Kate: Some people start [an eating disorder] by giving things up for Lent.
Vicky: I started by healthy eating . . . and like for breakfast I'd just eat fruit . . . Everyone drank Diet Coke but I just couldn't drink anything like that . . . I couldn't drink Diet Coke . . . I just thought it had loads of calories.
Kate: I didn't think about calories . . . I just thought about fat.
Vicky: I measured fat at first.
Kate: Yeah . . . I measured fat . . . I'd make sure that I didn't have like more than 5g of fat in a day . . . and then it went down to like no more than 1g.
(Fg)

The recontextualisation of the notion that 'fat kills' as positively sanctioned 'healthy eating' had seriously damaging consequences for these young people's health. In the view of one teacher:

I'm sure they were taught about healthy diets and unfortunately I think the emphasis is very often on low-fat diets . . . 'Don't eat too much fat, it's bad

for your heart' . . . etc. . . . 'Cholesterol . . . damages your blood vessels' . . .
and all the rest of it . . . [They] learn about that and they take that on board
and they don't realise that this is not to do with young people who are still
growing.

(Mrs Bailey, In)

This was clearly reflected in the experience of one of the young women:

Lara: Erm . . . I counted fat at the very start cos I didn't, like, have a clue about
calories . . . I didn't know what they were.
RA: Yeah . . . that's exactly what I did.
Lara: I counted fat but I did eat a very unhealthy diet and I was overweight when
I was younger and I just started out . . . and I think I just went really extreme
and just went to, like, salad and everything and I cut out, like, the meals
and had no fat and stuff.

(In)

Whose problem (and responsibility) is it, anyway?
Science talking morality, not science

Once a health problem is 'discovered', assigning responsibility for causes and
solutions forms the crux of public discourse (Lawrence, 2004: 58). As Gard
and Wright (2005: 6) have observed: 'very few of those who have announced
the "obesity epidemic"'s arrival have been satisfied with being mere messengers.
Most have also been unable to resist the temptation of claiming to know why it is
occurring and what we need to know about it.' *Super Size Me* and other media
contribute to these discourses in the quest to find a cause and solution to the obesity
epidemic. Spurlock explored whether food companies were solely to blame for
obesity and where personal responsibility stops and corporate responsibility
begins. This quest to attribute personal and corporate responsibility reflects wider
debates in obesity studies and health policy, often polarised disputes between those
who regard health as a matter of individual responsibility, lifestyle and behaviour
and those who consider the parts played by social and structural environments
(see Duncan, 2004: 178). Like the *JOTVS*, *Super Size Me* frames the problem of
obesity as a 'symptom of an unhealthy food and activity environment created,
either inadvertently or intentionally, by corporate and public policy' (Lawrence,
2004: 62). Blame is placed on the fast-food industry's emphasis on 'super-sizing'
everything. Fast-food culture has pervaded our society, including school cafeterias,
enticing people into 'risky' eating practices through marketing promotions, such
as McDonald's 'Happy Meal' for children. Thus, the film's narrative offers a
particular vision of the role of 'agency' in which there is nodding acknowledge-
ment of 'corporate responsibility' but 'health' is primarily an issue of morality and
individual responsibility (see Nettleton, 1997): 'We don't have to go there [fast-
food restaurants]. We can easily go into McDonald's and buy a salad but we *choose*
not to' (female member of public, *Super Size Me*). Healthy behaviour is presented

as and becomes 'a moral duty' and 'illness an individual moral failing' (Crawford, 1980: 365) based on what we choose to do. Echoes of these regulative codes resonated in the *JOTVS*, for example, as Oliver angrily vented his frustration on families who choose not to adhere to and support his ideals of eating and good food.

Am I to blame?

This notion of 'self-cultivation' is clearly reflected in the perspectives of the young people in our study, drawing upon liberal humanist ideas relating to individual 'control over his or her destiny'. Individuals are positioned inescapably in this discourse as 'best able to effect change to make his or her life "better"' (Nettleton, 1997: 208), with capacity for 'self-control, responsibility, rationality and enterprise' (*ibid.*: 214). In Klein's (1996: 22) view:

> In our culture, fat is evil. Eating it or wearing it, feeding it or bearing it is a sign of some moral deficiency. Aesthetically, physically and morally, fat is a badge of shame. A visible sign that in some areas of our life we have failed to be all we could be. An inescapable source of disappointment, of sadness and guilty self-contempt – of unrelenting shame.

These elemental tropes of popular culture, dangerously unmediated by appropriate concern for ages and stages of individual maturation or developmental needs, were reflected in teachers' and young people's attitudes and behaviour towards eating and food in school, as will become evident in subsequent chapters, where we refer to the viewpoints and opinions of the teachers and students who were involved in our research.

Spurlock's search for where corporate responsibility ends and individual responsibility begins sets the context for invoking what Halse (2007) refers to as 'bio-citizenship'. The sort of responsibility invoked in the film is not merely that individuals should be responsible for themselves but should look after themselves *for the sake of others*. As Halse points out, the discourse around BMI has a constitutive effect in championing a humanist ontology of the subject in which taking responsibility for ensuring one's weight falls within BMI norms is constituted as care for one's self *and* others and is fashioned into a social and ethical duty to wider society. Again, this ethic is reflected in the actions of teachers and the curriculum of schools:

RA: How did you feel when you had these 'healthy eating' lessons at school?
Jane: I think it made me a bit worse . . . There was the teacher . . . she was saying stuff to all the pupils like, 'Oh, you're all so lucky at the moment, you can eat like houses but you'll all be really fat when you're older if you carry on eating like this.'

(In)

A discourse of individualism is offered as the solution, where individuals are implicitly held personally responsible and accountable for the prevention of obesity and related health problems by knowing and avoiding relevant 'risk factors'. Spurlock's closing challenge is:

> If this ever-growing paradigm is going to shift, it's up to you. But if you decide to keep living this way, go ahead – over time you may find yourself getting as sick as I did and you may wind up here [image of hospital appears] or here [image of cemetery appears]. I guess the big question is: who do you want to see go first, you or them?

Such discourses invoke the sort of bio-citizenship which Halse (2007) describes. Spurlock (like Oliver) crafts critique into a moral obligation and responsibility not only for oneself but for the rest of the community in its fight against fast-food culture and some civic duty not to contribute to rising rates of obesity. Wallack and Lawrence's (2005) argument that there is insufficient public language through which to communicate *both* the structural nature of health problems *and* their solutions resonates with the way obesity and food issues are framed in *Super Size Me* and *JOTVS*. The sort of embodied individualism expressed in these extracts from them (and many other instances could be provided from other TV series: for example, and perhaps *par excellence*, Gillian McKeith's *You Are What You Eat*) makes it easier for people to imagine what one person might or might not do to be healthy compared with what society might collectively do to ensure health for its population.

    As with much media coverage of these issues, *JOTVS* and *Super Size Me* clearly adopt the position that the public needs to be 'better informed' about eating bad food and the 'obesity crisis'. Media seldom report biomedicine directly, instead adopting usually alarmist storylines to connect health promotion ideals and their implications for public health. Readers and viewers are assumed to be 'deficient', their knowledge unreliable, inadequate and 'profane', in the face of sufficient 'sacred' science. In *Super Size Me* expert voices were chosen on the basis of their ability to inform us about the 'facts' about obesity and fast-food culture and the 'science' behind food and health. The film draws upon a discourse which is, in many ways, 'comforting' because of the simplicity of the message – if you want to be healthy, remain or become thin (Campos, 2004). Like *JOTVS*, it raises a number of interesting questions about how 'public experts' are utilised in the construction of particular health discourses within the media, whose voices are heard or silenced as it locates and allocates blame:

> the contemporary citizen is increasingly attributed with responsibilities to ceaselessly maintain and improve her or his own health by using a whole range of measures. To do this she or he is increasingly expected to take note of and act upon the recommendations of a whole range of 'experts' and 'advisors' located in a range of diffuse institutional and cultural sites.
>
> (Bunton and Burrows, 1995: 208)

The 'educational' and psychological implications of popular pedagogies

Given the pervasiveness of such discourse in film and TV and their reproduction and endorsement by teachers and schools, it is hardly surprising that the young women in our study tended to construct narratives around their own bodies which reflected morally responsible, food- and diet-conscious, exercise-prone, 'neo-liberal' self-images. They felt that they were expected to be 'autonomous and flexible to negotiate, choose, succeed' (Walkerdine, 2003: 240) in myriad education and health contexts. It is equally unsurprising that their achievements were usually tempered by feelings of anxiety and depression, of never having been good enough. In both education and health matters, 'excellent' or 'elite' subjectivities were no sooner achieved than they were lost as standards shifted, leaving these young women in a state of liminality (see Chapter 7), living out expectancies they could never fulfil (Walkerdine *et al.*, 2001). As Lucey and Reay (2002: 351) suggest, for middle-class girls like these, constant striving for high attainment in neo-liberal education or health contexts, rather than engendering a sense of unproblematic confidence in their abilities, can produce a sense of never being adequate. With school discourse reflecting performance imperatives while, at the same time, giving overt and persistent attention to weight and shape ideals, it is also unsurprising that they recount experiences where their bodies were not only assessed against prescribed criteria in interactions over which they had no control, but put on public display, with horror:

> We used to have to get weighed in the class and that was terrible [. . .] It was to do with maths or something . . . and that was horrible . . . because then everybody knew your weight and then . . . a lot of the lads actually used to go on . . . and . . . you know . . . shouting out your weight in the class . . . things like that . . . that was terrible . . . really terrible.
>
> (Rebekah, In)

> I used to be overweight and I remember one time at school when the whole class got weighed and the teacher said, 'Oh, it's the big one,' and I was the heaviest in the year!
>
> (Lara, Pd)

In effect, they were subject to a form of liberal governance which produced particular affects of anxiety, stress and guilt, even though they were neither simply internalising performative, popular culture or school curricular messages nor reading them uncritically. Indeed, many recognised and resented their damaging effects:

> Food tech is a big problem because my teachers are always passing the message that fat is bad and that we all need to cut down, which isn't true because we are teenagers and we are growing. This message needs to be turned

around because it is not helpful for some people, that is all they need to convince them to stop eating.

(Vicky, Dd)

Vicky and others (see Chapter 4) showed both an acute awareness of and opposition to the social conditions of performative health cultures. They were aware of how popular culture sanctioned the authority of schools and teachers in endorsing 'body perfection codes', structures of meaning defining what size, shape, predisposition and demeanour bodies are and ought to be, as well as appropriate treatment, repair and restoration for those who do not meet these ideals (Evans and Davies, 2004). Vicky's experience was typical of that of many of our interviewees, where health was judged in terms of outward performances, such as not eating, exercising regularly and body appearance. As we will see, the co-option of media-articulated health concerns into pedagogical practice had placed these young people under constant surveillance, pressing them towards monitoring their bodies not through coercion but by facilitating *knowledge* about 'obesity'-related risks/issues and 'instructing' them on how to eat healthily, stay active and lose weight. Lara (see p. 75) felt objectified through public scrutiny and measurement of her body *and* was unable to express this discontent to her teacher. Instead, her response to this pedagogical encounter was to engage with extreme weight-loss practices in order to 'get her weight down quickly'.

Conclusion

We are concerned to illustrate how symbols relating to the body and how we are to think about either maintaining or restoring its 'health' enter into and encode the communicated content of popular culture transmitted through magazines, film and TV. We are equally concerned, however, with the decoding done by individuals, with how meanings, such as those drawn from popular culture, are 'interpreted and used in everyday life' (Fowles, 1996: xv; see also Kenway and Bullen, 2001), including school contexts. Critical studies of obesity discourse have centred on analyses of the media's use of text and imagery, the media message, in the discursive production of what has constituted a moral panic, the problem–resolution spin cycle that has characterised central governments' approaches towards education since the early 1980s. Their use of popular culture to signify affinity with a broad electoral base and as endorsement of health and green interests/agendas has been a particular concern. But rarely has the voice of popular pedagogy itself been adequately explored. We have highlighted the potential potency that this voice derives from its 'erotic' elements, particularly its desire to produce pleasure in search of a mass audience and profit, and the way it presented a promise of an idealised lifestyle, though unattainable for most. In effect, the voice created by popular culture creates a number of social and emotional anxieties, perhaps especially for those middle-class individuals who are expected to achieve its highest aspirations and ideals. Even where 'success', whether in education or health/weight terms, is achieved, the young women in our study report a constant sense of anxiety, failure and coping with such pressures via psychopathological narratives of extreme body modification. They use their bodies to signify both acceptance and rejection of contemporary cultures, to announce their distinction, while simultaneously stating corporeally that they do not and cannot endorse them (see Rich and Evans, forthcoming).

This chapter has also highlighted the importance of recognising the potential these media have for both sanctioning and perhaps mobilising new and innovative public discussions about obesity and weight-related issues. Conceivably they could provide new insight into the complexities of health and body (weight/health) issues. But *Super Size Me*, like other offerings in this genre, does not open up a meaningful 'debate' or engagement with the socio-cultural construction of obesity, food or weight issues. Instead, it sanctions a particularly reductive view of health as 'weight management' and diet as an issue of good or bad foods which becomes reflected in the policy and actions of teachers and pupils in schools. Understanding why popular culture and the knowledge it delivers might not be considered sufficient as a means of engaging the public in more meaningful dialogue about obesity will require a more culturally informed perspective on the ethics of health documentaries and their associated pedagogies. A greater sensitivity to the socio-cultural contexts of health and medicine is required. Miah (2005: 412) has argued, however, that scientists are 'most certainly the wrong kind of expert to use for ethical commentaries on science'; yet, in obesity discourse, this is precisely what occurs. He argues that advancing the methodological assumptions of public under-standing of science could be achieved through developing a public engagement with ethics. Obesity would be a particularly good subject area through which to do this for two key reasons: the relevant 'science' is replete with uncertainties and we frequently see 'well-known obesity scientists', whose tone would suggest otherwise, 'caught in the act' of speculation (Gard and Wright, 2005: 6); and while scientists tend to be experts who claim to be taking an objective, 'scientific' view, they construct a discourse laced with morality, ideology and science. They become the moral commentators on their own science, without having to reveal explicit moral or ethical positions. Could it be that a broader ethical and moral discussion about obesity may provide a more meaningful engagement for the public in a debate dominated by ethical posturing and attendant moral panic?

6 Solving the obesity crisis?

Health P/policy in totally pedagogised schools

Body pedagogies, P/policy and the pedagogic device

> Everyone at school's got, like, food issues . . . all the girls are always looking for, like, what's got the least fat and that . . . and people will comment on each other, like if someone has two chocolate bars, someone will say, like, 'Oh, haven't you had one already?' and stuff.
>
> (Tracey, In)

How are the voices of young people shaped, privileged or marginalised in the practices of education and schooling? How do pupils deal with the normalising expectations and requirements of performative culture and obesity discourse? Can they evade, accommodate or recontextualise relentless and penetrating surveillance of their bodies in school time and space? If we are to begin to understand such processes we need to press beyond analyses of the intrinsic content of obesity 'messages' to consider 'the voice' of education itself and how it is shaped by the *pedagogic device* (see Figure 1, p. 23): 'a grammar for producing specialised messages, realisations, a grammar which regulates what it processes: a grammar which orders and positions and yet contains the potential of its own transformation' (Bernstein, 1990: 190). 'Obesity discourse' nurtures a language, grammar and syntax with regulative and instructional principles and codes which define thought and action; or, in Bernstein's terms, a 'meaning potential' for 'health' largely in terms of weight, size and shape, where the solution to 'problems' is a matter of weight loss through taking more exercise and eating less food. This language relates to global trends and issues shaped and formed through contemporary policy and pedagogies on education and health and embodied in and voiced through the actions of young people in and outside schools. Focusing on these relationships, we can demonstrate how 'the voice' of health/education policy articulated through a language of 'performativity' creates a culture which inadvertently endorses actions (such as those voiced by Tracey, above) that are damaging for some young people's education and for their health.

Schools as totally pedagogised micro-societies (TPMS)

We live in a 'knowledge economy' (Hargreaves, 2003) in which schools are expected to nurture and endorse particular 'corporeal orientations', ascribing value, meaning and potential to 'the body' in time, place and space. Such processes are not arbitrary but reflect wider national and global socio-economic trends. In contemporary culture they increasingly celebrate the particular virtues of 'flexible identities' manifested in aspects of 'performance' and 'corporeal perfection'. The latter is usually defined in terms of 'the slender ideal', linking personal, embodied subjectivities to global economic trends. As we will see below, 'knowledge economy' expectations relating to the body and health enter schools neither straightforwardly nor only through the perspectives and actions of individuals. They are given voice through two forms of policy: 'formal', state-sanctioned, usually legislated education *Policy*; and 'informal', mainly medical and health institution-based, state-'approved' but non-legislated, pseudo *policy* initiatives, often merely reflecting expectations and pressures recontextualised by the popular media, for example, relating to diets and exercise levels (Evans *et al.*, 2008). Together, these P/policies determine what is to count within formal education as official or 'sacred' health knowledge, what it is correct to believe and know about health matters as related by relevant health sciences, as well as increasingly encoding other aspects of school life, in effect making 'pedagogy' everyone's concern, everywhere. These processes are relentless and inescapable, and they define the nature of pedagogical activity in the totally pedagogised micro-societies (TPMS) which schools have become.

Like all other dimensions of educational systems, both pedagogy and teachers' work are altered by changes that occur outside schools, sometimes on a global scale. In our knowledge-driven economies, technological revolutions, the development of communication systems and changes in production processes and work organisation are just some of the factors that potentially alter not only what is taught but how and where teaching occurs, as Hargreaves (2003) and Bonal and Rambla (2003) have pointed out. The teaching profession itself is transformed in such processes, as are the structures of educational messages. Bonal and Rambla have argued, for example, that 'new teachers' are more likely to become knowledge managers than knowledge experts. They must be as capable of informing children and young people how to 'access' knowledge, including 'physical' knowledge, both in and outside school, as they are of imbuing them with specific competences and skills during the school day. For example, in the language of the QCA (2007), young people must 'follow pathways to other activities in and beyond school' and teachers must be capable of identifying different and diverse student capabilities and abilities and willing to update their knowledge constantly to cope with frequent and rapid changes in society. Systems of audit and accountability, for example, in the UK through Ofsted, Estyn (the school inspection service in Wales) and the Teacher Development Agency, are put in place to monitor their performances. Schools continue to be held responsible not just for educating future workers' 'abilities' but for socialising them as good citizens. They are not only expected to have explicit roles in the transmission of values and attitudes (Bonal and Rambla, 2003: 171) but to contrive everyday arrangements that engender what students ought to and should achieve by way of an 'embodied presence' as preparation for work and 'healthy living'. In the UK, as elsewhere, a curriculum dealing with 'citizenship' or personal and social education (PSE) – which, indicatively, became personal, social, health and economic education (PSHEE), in the recent secondary school curriculum review (QCA, 2007) – as preparation for working life has become an increasingly officially privileged curricular concern.

On the demand side, recent work in the UK by Brown and his colleagues has focused on the graduate labour market, specifically on what employers seek in graduate trainees and the processes by which companies and corporations select them from the graduate 'pool' (Brown and Hesketh, 2004; Smetherham, 2004). Employers now place value on 'soft skills' alongside conventional degree qualifications. 'Soft skills' in this context comprise good communication, ease of rapport with others and capacities for mediation and negotiation. Increasingly, they have also come to mean particular body orientations in which correct size, shape and 'appearance' are credentials for certain jobs (Fikkan and Rothblum, 2005). From a Bernsteinian perspective, these are qualities strongly associated with and tacitly acquired through the 'invisible pedagogy' that characterises 'new' middle-class family interactions. Employers value these manifest qualities because graduates are taken not only to represent but literally to embody 'the face' of the company and its health and vibrancy in the wider world. It is perhaps no surprise in this respect, then, that in the UK subjects such as PE and sport in secondary schools[1] and sports science in universities have flourished in recent years (Griggs and Wheeler, 2006). They are held to produce a particular form of cultural capital, a new form of 'the rounded individual', through emphases on the production of particular corporeal dispositions or orientations. In essence, PE and sport, along with other subjects delivering 'soft skills', such as PSHEE and citizenship education, have become part of the ethic of 'trainability' (Bernstein, 2001). Moreover, these processes are also enacted across a variety of sites in and outside schools and are reflected in the language of P/policy on 'health'.

Performativity and body pedagogies in TPMS

In almost his last published work Bernstein (2001) alluded to the second emergence of what he referred to as the 'totally pedagogised society' (TPS). In such contexts, pedagogy not only pervades every aspect of life (for example, media websites, TV, family, playgrounds, doctors' surgeries, as well as school classrooms) but features throughout one's lifetime. Individuals are expected to 'work on' or refashion themselves routinely and relentlessly, or be 'worked on' or refashioned by others in the interests of pre- or proscribed ideals (for example, those relating to employment or health). A range of expertise across a variety of sites is made available, seemingly to help the public avoid the 'risks' of modern-day living and achieve what they are expected to be: independent, successful and 'healthy', with the last of these usually misrecognised in Western cultures as 'being thin'. Hence, in the UK, we are bombarded with information and advice on what to eat, how to exercise, where to live, what clothes to wear and what weight we should be, with the last of these dictated from early life by the World Health Organisation's new guidelines on infant weight scales (BBC News, 2006). Since 2005, in line with these guidelines, pupils in primary school reception classes (age four–five) and Year 6 (age ten) have been weighed and measured.

Bernstein argued that the emergence of the TPS related to the nature of postmodern economies in which knowledge was relatively fluid and ephemeral, giving rise to labour processes where long-term 'careers' are replaced by short-term 'jobs' (Bonal and Rambla, 2003). In such contexts, TPS emerges as a crucial regulator of everyday experience, translating uncertainty, risk and precariousness into a form of socialisation characterised by endless learning and trainability. Schools remain central to this process, occupying around 15,000 hours of a child's time during their compulsory, student careers between the ages of five and sixteen in the UK but only as one among many sites of pedagogical activity (see Figure 1, p. 23). They tend to become, as Bonal and Rambla (*ibid.*: 169) put it, closely paraphrasing Bernstein, focused upon 'trainability': that is, the 'ability to profit from continuous pedagogic reformations and so cope with the new requirements of work and life . . . the key concept and mechanism through which the TPS emerges'. Individuals have to be able to act on new knowledge and be prepared to 'reform themselves' endlessly to meet the new and fast-changing needs of capital: '"Trainability" entails a continuous disposition of the subject to be trained for the requirements of his/her entire life . . . The acquirer never knows enough and never will be able to develop enough abilities to learn' (*ibid.*: 174). It is hardly surprising that in such contexts the dominant pedagogical model focuses on 'performance', for knowledge – which is volatile, changes fast and does not produce a sense of certainty in the acquirer but has to be closely related to specific outputs, while pedagogy has to be 'generic'. These necessities, it is claimed, are colonising formal educational policies and school practices, transforming teachers' work and identities.[2] We suggest it is also reflected in the actions and attitudes of some children and young people towards their bodies, in and outside schools. In such contexts accountability, competition and constant comparison (with reference, for example, to performance targets, test scores or exam league tables) have become the *lingua franca* of this new discourse of power, creating a 'performative society' (Ball, 2004a) that constantly demands that teachers and students display evidence of a willingness to work on themselves or their institutions to meet criteria and standards of education and health set elsewhere and over which they have little or no control (see Chapter 7). The effects are profound and potentially deeply psychologically damaging for both teachers *and* students who are involved in processes of being constantly assessed and asked to strive for better grades, better shapes and weights, to reach 'gold standards' that are no sooner achieved than they become denigrated or changed (Carlyle and Woods, 2002). This discourse plays its part, as Ball (2004a: 144) puts it, in 'making us up', producing new modes of description and new possibilities for action and despair as new social identities are created. It also impacts upon social relations in schooling where 'authentic relationships' are replaced by ones which are more judgemental; people are valued for their productivity or performances alone. A culture is created that lends itself to alienation of the self as people are constantly required to make themselves different and distinct through 'micro-practices of representation' judgement and comparison: for example, through academic performance, or what they eat, or how they exercise, or what they weigh. While we will say more of how these processes are relayed through the academic culture of schools to impact upon the lives of young people in the next chapter, here we focus on how a culture of performativity has infused and encoded P/policies on health education in schools.

Health discourse in performative culture

'Educational texts' are not the only 'performative texts' which confront teachers and students and 'increasingly deform practices in schools' (Ball, 2004a: 143). Indeed, focusing only on official 'education Policy' can distract us from the significance of other codes and their pedagogical modalities, elsewhere referred to as 'perfection codes' (Evans and Davies, 2004), which find their ways into health contexts in schools. These, as we saw in Chapter 3, tend to have their social bases outside formal education, for example, in medical and health fields. Their pedagogic modalities (body pedagogies) are shaped largely independently of both educational official and pedagogical recontextualising fields, for example, by agencies such as the World Health Organisation and, in the UK, the British Heart Foundation. Increasingly, however, leading figures ('experts') from the world of health have been successfully co-opted or incorporated into the state apparatus to advise on, among other things, both the form and content of PE and health education and other practices (e.g., diets and exercise levels) in schools.[3]

In the UK, health iterations/recommendations rarely progress straightforwardly into schools in the form of 'Policy' but tend, initially at least, to remain 'authoritative prescriptions' or 'frameworks of expectation' produced by analyses of what are taken to be the underlying features necessary for achievement of physical, psychological, social and intellectual health or 'better lifestyles' in contemporary society. Such messages tend, first, to be recontextualised through media, such as websites, TV and newspapers, saturating popular culture before entering schools either as government Policy legislation or as policy initiatives taken by schools themselves or induced by central government in response to health concerns (see Chapter 5). Such initiatives taken by schools themselves, frequently prior to or alongside more formal government Policy legislation, often follow agendas set outside the educational establishment. Discourse around obesity is an obvious example (Gard and Wright, 2005; Burrows and Wright, 2004a). In the UK the 'expertise' of high-profile celebrity figures (for example, chefs, dieticians and fitness gurus) has been called on to set expectations as to how life in schools, families and among others in contact with students or children can be altered or re-engineered to ensure that bodies are refashioned into what they ought to be. At one level, some schools have acted independently in response to such concerns, for example, by improving lunch menus. At another, central government has sought joint action from the Department of Health (DoH) and the Department for Education and Skills (DfES) to address health matters through Policy which affects not just the formal curriculum but the 'whole environment' of schools. For example, a National Healthy Schools Programme (NHSP) was introduced in 1999, with new, 'more rigorous' guidelines issued in 2005 (DoH, 2005a), to address 'pressing health concerns'. Initially, it served as a vehicle to support delivery of personal, social and health education (PSHE), a formal curricular element and to 'engage staff, pupils, governors, parents and the wider community in a whole school approach to educational achievement, health and emotional well being' (teachernet, 2006). 'Healthy schools' are now expected to monitor almost every aspect of pupils' lives, including 'sex and relationships education', drug education, healthy eating, physical activity, health and well-being. Such schools, for example, will have 'meals, vending machines and tuck shop facilities that are nutritious and healthy and meet or exceed national standards'; will monitor pupils' 'menus and food choices to inform policy development and provision'; and will 'consult pupils on food choices through the school day' (DoH, 2005: 8). Moreover, since 2005, such initiatives have been evaluated and 'supported' in England through official Ofsted school inspections that report on the contribution every school makes to specified 'outcomes' relating to education and health.

Such P/policies not only enter into and are intended to define the cultural fabric of schools 'as a whole' – that is to say, to create a totally pedagogised micro-society – but their 'perfection codes' are inescapably 'linked to the incipient madness of the requirements of performativity' (Ball, 2004a: 147). They intersect with ideologies, principles and policies that are already *in situ*, according to the established grammar given by the pedagogic device. Its assessment arrangements now require schools to provide visible 'evidence' in core PSHE themes of healthy eating, physical activity and emotional health and well-being, while 'using a whole school approach involving the whole school community' (DoH, 2005: 4). This discourse enjoins schools to work at one of 'three levels'. At the highest, level 3, schools will have demonstrated 'a more intensive level of involvement by having undertaken a process of auditing, target setting and action planning'. Again, a language of performativity pervades this text, as it continues:

> The impact of activities is assessed through school monitoring and evaluation, with a particular focus on pupils' learning outcomes . . . [I]n order to achieve national consistency at level 3, schools are expected to fulfil specific criteria drawn from the NHSS and have evidence of the impact of development work for each criterion. This requirement is in line with current practice in schools where evidence is collected for celebration of success through the local healthy schools programme. The national evaluation of the NHSS, which is underway, will build on these criteria to provide more refined indicators for the future.
>
> (teachernet, 2006)

Schools might achieve level 3 involvement when there is a range of 'evidence of impact', demonstrating that all of the criteria have been met. This culture not only pervades activities across many sites inside schools but reaches across the sector. It is reported that 'since the final rounds of accreditation were attained in April 2002, Local Education Authority Participation in the NHSS programme has reached 100 per cent'. In effect:

> over 14,000 schools are taking part in the healthy schools scheme at level 2 and 8,000 are working intensively at level 3 to achieve the standard. Half of these schools serve deprived areas [. . .] All schools in England with 20 per cent or more free school meal entitlement should be recruited to the programme by 2006.
>
> (teachernet, 2006)

Although many of these initiatives enter schools under the guise of liberal practice, they reify performative culture and are constructed within a language of putatively evidence-based activity and accountability, claiming comparative measures as to whether healthy behaviours prevail. As with the recent Policy initiative to weigh and measure all primary schoolchildren at age four and ten, no teacher, pupil or parent can escape surveillance or regulation of their willingness and ability to address what are defined as pressing health concerns. Perfection codes are thus reflected in pedagogical activity across a range of sites and, as with performance codes, they position the body as being in deficit, unfinished or at risk and in need of rescue from influences over which individuals or populations have ever less control. Focus is directed to outside school experience and lifestyles generally in terms of future perspectives as to what could or is to be achieved, given the 'right' embodied capacities in terms of actions and attitudes towards health (Evans and Davies, 2004, 2008). For this reason, they are best characterised as 'body-centred perfection codes' generating particular body 'policies' and body pedagogies, actions designed to foster particular corporeal orientations to one's own and others' bodies in time, place and space.

They enter the school system through P/policies which not only affect the formal curriculum but prescribe young people's lifestyle choices. For example, on 14 May 2006, under the headline 'Schools Fight Fat with Fingerprinting', *Times Online* reported a UK initiative taken by schools to address growing obesity concerns, claiming that: 'Unhealthy habits could be banished as pupils have their fingers scanned at the dinner queues . . . Schools are increasingly using fingerprint techniques . . . in an attempt to speed up service and promote healthy eating.' The concerns of civil liberty groups over the legality and potential misuse of such biometric data were ignored as teachers purportedly warmly welcomed the initiative because 'it would allow schools to pass on information about what pupils were eating to parents. The aim was to promote more healthy eating.' As we have pointed out, parents and teachers were putatively united, it seems, in the raging war against 'obesity disease'. Armed with modern technology, they would together take concerted, radical action to monitor and regulate their children's/pupils' behaviour, rein in and rehabilitate their bad eating habits and bring food suppliers, including parents, under closer scrutiny and control. Placing young people under such surveillance presses them towards monitoring their bodies not through coercion but by facilitating 'knowledge' about 'obesity'-related risks/issues and 'instructing' them on how to eat healthily, stay active and lose weight. These become ubiquitous when expressed within a 'totally pedagogised society', where methods to evaluate, monitor and survey the body are encouraged across a range of sites, not only schools but popular media, new technologies and health organisations. In school these body pedagogies construct particular social meanings which influence young people's identities not only in relation to health but in the academic performance they are expected to display and achieve, as the voices of the young people quoted below highlight.

Body pedagogies in a TPMS

It is hardly surprising, then, that the young people in our study constructed their identities and subjectivities – more specifically, their health and illness – through the language of performativity and the health discourses that dominate contemporary culture and feature in their school experience. They got to know about their bodies and health not only through the language of 'experts', such as health educators and teachers in schools but through P/policy-created official curricular content and informal interaction and discourse. Although, in a variety of school contexts they all tended to speak with a single voice of their schools transmitting 'body perfection codes', structures of meaning defining body size, shape, predisposition and demeanour and how, for those who do not meet these ideals, treatment, repair and restoration were provided. While relatively few were impelled to take the dramatic actions of these young people they vividly revealed features of a TPMS which are rapidly on the increase across Western countries (Grogan, 1999) and generate increasing levels of body disaffection and dissatisfaction, to which all are subject.

These girls made repeated reference either to a culture of intensified expectations endemic in schools or their expression in specific subjects. For example, Ellie and Lydia commented that they had lost weight in order to receive more recognition from their PE teachers and to move into higher-grade sports teams. They perceived that PE teachers equated 'thin' not just with being 'healthy' but as an indication of their commitment both to the subject matter and the aim of losing weight. Claire, too, had found PE problematic: 'In PE they used to tell us not to be lazy and called people lazy if they thought they weren't trying hard enough' (Claire, In). Mia (In) was encouraged by her swimming coach to lose weight so that she 'would move faster through the water'. She reported that problems over competition had led her to change schools and that in her new swimming team she was able to progress into the 'top lane' (i.e., she was among the best swimmers). As this achievement coincided with reaching her lowest weight, she was able to meet simultaneously the symbiotic expectations of 'academic performance' and body perfection codes.

Emphasis on competition and ever rising, never attainable, perfect academic states was a major concern for these young women (see Chapter 7), with teachers such as Mr Sheldon (at the centre where they were now 'recovering') tending to see an increase in their numbers during examination periods:

> To be honest around this time we usually have an influx of students who are doing exams . . . [A]t the moment I've only got one who's booked in to do GCSEs here . . . but by the end of next month I guarantee there'll be four or five [. . .] every year's the same. I mean, I start off by not having many who are at the exam age or they're not taking GCSEs, . . . and then all of a sudden there are four or five, and the one year I had ten, eleven in here doing exams.
>
> (Mr Sheldon, In)

He was equally aware that emphasis placed on performativity in terms of achieving exam results had more to do with establishing and protecting the reputations and interests of schools than meeting educational needs and the interests of students:

> Yes, they are . . . I think a lot of schools they . . . they have errr . . . because there are tables and errr . . . of the expectations for good passes and the further up the national table it tends to put the teachers under pressure and also the students under pressure to gain . . . you know . . . the best that they can out of exams and classes and whether they've got A*s and As and . . . there is quite a lot of pressure . . . especially if the students are very bright, because we get an awful lot of students here who are on the A axis and not the Bs and the Cs and the Ds.
>
> (Mr Sheldon, In)

Several young women during focus group discussions, at interview and in diary and poster presentations reported that there was pressure in subjects such as PE, health and PSE and that they were subject to surveillance and the normalising effects of biopower through social relationships in corridors, at play times, during lunch breaks and in interactions and iterations among peers generally in and outside schools. This was reflected in the experience of the girls quoted below:

> The pressure to look perfect took over your study work . . . everyone used to look at you . . . you wouldn't go to school if you had a spot.
>
> (Tracey, In)

Vicky: Some girls, when I was like at my lowest weight . . . one girl said to me, 'You look really good.'

Kate: All my friends said to me, 'Oh God, you've lost so much weight, you look well good!' and 'You look fantastic' . . . and I was like, 'Yeah, thanks . . . I know!' . . . cos I thought I looked good.

Lara: You get a lot of like 'Oh, you've lost weight' and then you feel like you can't put it back on cos they'll like notice it . . . d'you know what I mean?

(Fg)

In such a culture school lunchtimes and 'free time' become hugely problematic, especially for girls. Lunchtimes, in particular, are virulent environments, with girls surveying their own and others' behaviour. As several girls recalled during focus group discussions:

RA: Anything at school that you felt influenced you?
Anne: Yeah . . . people not really eating properly, which made me think, 'Hold on . . . what am I doing . . . I'm eating so much more than them.'
Vicky: I was like that too! [Most people in the group agree] . . . Yeah . . . some other people weren't eating anything . . . Not many people were eating like a proper lunch so there was no way I was going to [. . .]
Kate: At my school . . . all the girls have like a tiny, tiny little bread roll when there's, like, a big variety of stuff and they just go and get one tiny little bread roll . . . It's like that big [indicates with her hand] . . . little bread roll and that's it . . . or nothing.
RA: Did many people feel like that then, that people weren't eating a proper lunch?
Lara: I did, but . . .
Vicky: My friends didn't eat their lunch at school, though . . .
Lara: I started, like, not eating and then, like, everyone else did too . . . Well, not like everyone else, but a lot of people did and that made me feel like I couldn't start eating it again . . . cos . . . when I was, like, trying to get better and that . . . no one else ate it then . . . so I didn't want to be the only one starting eating it again.

These young people drew on the 'moral' authority of governmental or health agency expertise, advice and information: for example, Ruth referred to 'healthy eating' to rationalise and guide her own actions towards food, first normalising then pathologising the behaviour that made her ill. Soon, the only diet worth following was no diet at all. Young people engage in these 'appropriate' behaviours not just in pursuit of 'health' but to achieve status and value in the eyes of peers, teachers and friends. They know that achieving the correct size and shape takes time but they provide markers of distinction as to how disciplined and 'good' they have become. Their quality and value is defined through their relationships with food, diet and exercise. As we have already seen in Chapter 5, performative culture is also reflected and endorsed in environments outside schools, such as TV, websites and information in doctors' surgeries. For some of the girls, magazines, TV and sometimes family life provided further endorsement of their health knowledge and behaviour. In the last of these, well-intentioned parents reconstituted 'appropriate' public discourse concerning the 'right' attitudes towards weight, diet and food, sometimes with dire health consequences, as related by Kate, Vicky and Claire:

Kate: OK . . . well . . . before . . . when I was happy with how I looked . . . I wasn't overweight or anything . . . I was like happy . . . and then like my dad said [. . .] he was gonna take me, my brother and my two sisters on holiday, and he said . . . he told us to all lose weight for the holiday so we'd look good in our swimwear . . . So me and my little sister we made a diet thing . . . we had to stick to that, we had to eat . . . like it was no chocolate or anything . . . and then I just took it too far cos, like . . . my Dad said . . . 'You could do with losing a bit of weight' . . . and then, like . . . when I went to school, like . . . and I'm used to things, like . . . when I went before all my friends were, like, skinny and I'm not . . . I never used to think that at all.

Vicky: Neither did I . . .

Kate: And then I just started thinking that and looking . . . and then I wouldn't be able to walk past a window or a mirror without looking in it and thinking, 'Oh my God' . . . So that's really all my dad's fault.

(Fg)

Claire: Erm . . . well . . . my mum used to go to Weight Watchers and then, like, she always said what was healthy and I used to read loads of magazines and on the telly it was, like, 'Eat lots of fruit and vegetables, eat five portions a day.'

RA: Yeah.

Claire: And then . . . I knew that, like, chips and burgers were fatty and crisps and chocolate and so anything . . . I think anything that you like is, like . . . bad, and things that are, like, boring are good.

(In)

A cursory reading of this data might inadvertently lead us to conclude that these young people were simply dupes, or their problems merely discursive reflections of pressures endemic in society and schools. But it is clear that they neither simply read nor internalised these messages uncritically, or merely 'cognitively', through disembodied 'knower structures', the intellectual schemas into which they have been socialised by virtue of their culture and their class. Rather, they were mediated by their flesh and blood, developing bodies, by chemistries, biologies and physiologies. These are punctuated by levels of maturation, the grammar and syntax of their 'textured feelings' influenced, if not determined, by their subcultural location in a specific time and space. Time and again these young people locate their difficulties viscerally and always relationally in their antecedent experiences of fast-changing, sometimes awkward, less than 'perfect' bodies, located among their teachers and peers:

When I started secondary school I'd, like . . . I'd started sort of . . . puberty quite early I'd say cos, erm . . . I started getting acne and stuff [. . .] Nobody had really mentioned anything about it before at primary school but when I went to secondary school . . . a couple of the lads started picking on me.

(Amanda, In)

When I was at school I was, like, bullied loads . . . like all through my school . . . so I just thought I was, like, crap basically . . . I thought . . . erm . . . I thought cos people didn't like me for who I was then there must be something wrong with me, so I thought that anyway I could, like, change myself . . . I thought of all the things I could change about myself . . . I thought, 'Well, I know one thing which I could change and would see results in is, like . . . my figure.'

(Claire, In)

I had started to develop much quicker than everyone else and I was interested in lads. All the girls turned against me and started calling me a slag and I felt like I had to live up to it.

(Lara, In)

Yeah, cos, like, I hit puberty early so I was always taller and, like . . . naturally bigger than everyone else . . . so that was always an issue cos you always feel like . . . out of it . . . you know? . . . with all your friends still in, like, really small clothes and stuff like that [. . .] So that was a major factor.

(Rebekah, In)

And at my new school I do remember, like, being really upset because . . . I, like . . . had a growth spurt and I got quite a bit bigger than what I was [. . .] and I thought . . . 'I have to cut down a bit' and then I just went to, like, healthy eating over the summer.

(Vicky, In)

Their changing bodies, over which they had little or no control, were inescapably subjected to both their own and others' evaluative gazes at home, at leisure and amid the pressures of totally pedagogised schools. Avoiding the pain of being 'othered', made to feel different, less worthy and excluded, by engaging in radical body modification involving excessive exercise and eating little or no food, experiencing the joy of achieving the distinction of 'thin' beyond the slender ideal, became, for some, a perfectly rational, morally acceptable goal.

Moralising and normalising behaviour

For many of these young women, escaping the normalising effects of techniques of biopower associated with obesity seemed inconceivable. 'Health education' had not only pervaded every aspect of their lives but had invoked social relations, sanctioned by the moral authority of 'obesity discourse', in which their opinions, interests and expertise were, in their view, patently ignored (for example, see Rebekah's comments on p. 107). The young women we interviewed highlighted powerful ways in which health discourse relating to exercise, food, diet and body size endorsed outside schools was taken up within school cultures with powerful effect, not only on the social relations of schooling but on individuals' developing sense of well-being and self. But, as we shall see in Chapter 7, it was a fragile self, a delicate identity, because the knowledge on which it was based was also fragile and ephemeral, exciting feelings of always being in pursuit of the 'right' behaviour and the right knowledge but of never achieving or being in control of them. Particular body shapes were recognised as being of high status and value but unattainable, so some were unable to recognise themselves as having a body and 'self' of any value at all. However, far from being cultural dopes, their radical actions were often intended to subvert performative culture. Shedding weight was a way of saying, 'Now I have "no body", I am in control, see me as a person, for who I really am.' They had few other mechanisms or opportunities to voice or display their deep dissatisfaction and discontent within the performative 'health' cultures of schools.

Clearly, the pressure wrought through P/policies and their associated pedagogies to obtain the right body size/shape was not simply about being healthy but carried moral characterisations of the obese or overweight as lazy, self-indulgent and greedy. The corollary of this (see Evans *et al.*, 2004c) was that control, virtue and goodness were to be found in slenderness and the processes of becoming thin. These behaviours were endorsed and legitimised within a culture of performativity or, more specifically, 'trainability', that prevailed in their schools, placing responsibility upon them as individuals to accept that correct diet, involvement in physical activity and the pursuit of 'perfection' academically were moral as well as corporeal obligations. Given the social sanctions that went with this discourse, including the bullying, stigma and labelling these girls mentioned, particularly being defined by their peers as 'fat', it was hardly surprising that many not only took drastic action to lose weight but became seriously depressed, as well as physically ill:

> I was always unhappy with the way I looked . . . I thought I was fat . . . I also got told I was fat. But it wasn't what people said to me that made me diet. I decided to go on a normal healthy diet. I would still have a chocolate bar here and there but just not so much. I was trying to cut down on high-fat foods and then, within a few weeks, I was only eating small amounts of salad during the day. Many people noticed my weight loss and told me I was skinny, but I didn't listen. I thought I looked good . . . I wasn't fat any more.
>
> (Kate, Pd)

While such narratives may underscore increasing levels of body disaffection, dissatisfaction with one's body is not necessarily an antecedent to ill health. Indeed, without contradiction, it may be a 'normal pathology'. Most people who are dissatisfied with their body do not go on to become ill for that reason, just as not everyone who is dangerously thin has become so because of the influence of popular media's affection for slender body ideals. Of course, we need to distinguish between corporeal dissatisfaction which may be a normative condition in all societies, at all times, in all places and disorder which may damage people's health. But it is here that studies of people who are struggling with serious 'body issues', such as anorexia and morbid obesity, seem so relevant. The voices of these young women illustrate that reducing analysis of body disaffection and disorder to the study of any single discourse (for example, 'healthism' or 'weightism'), with or without consideration of the pedagogic and corporeal devices, will, at best, provide only partial explanations of the conditions that may lead to alienation and ill health; at worst, it may obfuscate other, more damaging conditions of people's lives (Bryant-Waugh, 2000). High among such conditions are the social relations and knowledge hierarchies induced by performative culture in totally pedagogised schools.

7 Class, control and embodiment
What schools do to middle-class girls

Middle-class matters

> My Pressured Life. Big, trapped, 'live the dream', stress, work addict, get fit, exercise addict, I hate my figure, think, calorie counter, stand out, weight watchers, pushover, diet, beauty, changing, secrets, run away.
>
> (Amanda, Pd)

We began this book with reference to the social-class dimensions of obesity discourse, highlighting the way in which media coverage of obesity implicitly vilifies an overgeneralised, overworked and much maligned social category, 'the working class'. This 'category' purportedly acts irresponsibly towards health, providing 'bad food', 'bad parenting' and too little opportunity for good, clean, healthy living. Such discourse blames as it individualises, hiding complex structural factors like poor housing and income levels and government inaction on planning and provision that underlie social-class differences in health and longevity. In obesity discourse 'fat' or 'overweight' is rarely considered proxy for conditions, over which individuals may have little or no control, that blight working-class lives. We cannot in this book deal with the complexities of class/health issues but we do want to touch on some relationships that are either obfuscated or misrecognised in obesity discourse, particularly between popular culture, formal education and 'the middle class'. The last of these is relatively underexplored in sociological and educational research, often a 'shadowy and unsatisfactory presence' in much of the literature on sociology of education and pedagogy: 'It hovers in the background against which the perspectives and experiences of the working class have been contrasted' (Power and Whitty, 2002: 596). There are good reasons for this, given the stubborn persistence of social-class inequalities in education, employment, wealth and health, in the UK and elsewhere (see Butler and Savage, 1995; Ball, 2003a).[1] However, if nothing else, the voices of the young people reported throughout this book offer a salutary reminder that middle-class children also bleed; they are not always affirmed by pedagogic processes but may fail, feel alienated, neglected, used and damaged.

We want to elaborate on the ways in which the social trends outlined in Chapters 5 and 6 relating to 'the body' and health generate and intersect with what we have referred to as *performance* and *perfection* codes (Evans and Davies, 2004, following Bernstein, 2000b). These create conditions of schoolwork that, while increasingly difficult for many students, may be particularly problematic for 'middle-class' girls. Their multiple 'effects', which form pressures around health, status, control and the body, are those within which Amanda felt 'trapped'. Given both the symbolic and material value attributed to education in middle-class households, their children may be even more vulnerable to adverse school experiences than their working-class counterparts (Giddens, 1973). They are much less likely to be given opportunity through either personal 'choice' or academic design (school-induced 'failure') to leave the system early (at sixteen rather than eighteen in the UK). Some vulnerable few have to endure conditions which are not merely difficult but may be deeply damaging to their identities and health, particularly when coincident with other, problematic features of their lives.

Learning to be hungry

> I don't think that school caused my anorexia because there were a lot of issues at home and things, but I think it probably contributed to it because of the things that happened there.
>
> (Karen, Ic)

Anorexia nervosa, like all other eating disorders, is an extremely complex condition, variously understood and much debated across the disciplines of psychiatry, medicine, psychology, biology, sociology and epidemiology, whose sophistication would be difficult to overstate (see Lask and Bryant-Waugh, 2000). However, in Chapter 2 we argued that anorectic and other disordered eating behaviours and experiences have tended to be viewed both in the popular media and in much of the mainstream academic press as pathological conditions distinctly different from 'normal' and 'healthy' experiences and practices of non-anorexic women and girls (see also Malson, 1998). As such, they become separated from their social context and their everyday experiences. Hence, from a mainstream perspective, the object of enquiry is often essentially 'the disorder' – for example, the 'anorexia' – not the varied, complex and socially conceptualised experiences of individual girls and women who have been diagnosed as 'anorexic'. Previous chapters have announced our departure from these more traditional, pathological perspectives to reveal an emerging theoretical position on narratives of disordered eating in relation to education. The voices reported below prompt us again to reconsider the interplay between 'the body', power, knowledge and (ill) health within schools in relation to the aetiology and development of eating disorders, in this case anorexia nervosa. Their narratives challenge accounts of the misuse of food and exercise that lean over-heavily on either inherent, individual traits ('perfectionism') or external social factors celebrating the 'slender ideal' that predispose or motivate individuals. In the case of anorexia the 'trait' is usually defined as psychological, the need to escape from psychological problems that individuals cannot face, or the 'desire' to achieve 'perfection' or regain control.

However, such a view cannot adequately account for self-starvation or disordered eating, conditions where 'deviant' motives and activity develop in the course of experience, involving processes in which biology (physical development/ maturation) and culture inevitably collide. One has to *learn to become anorectic*, such that, as Becker (1971: 141) classically illustrated with reference to other forms of aberrant behaviour, 'instead of the deviant motives leading to the deviant behaviour, it is the other way around; the deviant behaviour in time produces the deviant motivation'. Vague impulses and desires – for example, the desire to get thin or to regain control – are transformed into definite patterns of behaviour and become part of the individual's 'lifestyle'. This transformation is not arbitrary but given shape, form and direction by the workings of the corporeal device as it intersects with and is given expression in the cultures and pedagogies of schools.

As we pointed out in Chapter 2 the complexity of this process belies the image presented in popular culture of eating disorders as a 'transitory, self inflicted problem developed by young women lost in their world of fashion and calorie restricting' (Katzman and Lee, 1997: 389). This approach to disordered eating perpetuates a 'belittling stereotype' masking more immediate and complex concerns experienced particularly by young women, not least within schools. Locating eating disorders only in a 'cult of slenderness' diminishes the complexities of gendered, embodied experiences, the ways in which power is enacted in social relations and the sense of distinction that can be derived from achieving identity as 'an anorexic'. At the same time, we do have to consider how media imagery and obesity discourse find their way into the socio-cultural fabric of schools and specific subject areas, as well as other cultural terrain (Pronger, 2002), acknowledging that these cultural conditions construct and legitimise particular body images and forms of 'body work'. School culture and peer pressures can intersect to create conditions that make individuals' relationships with food problematic, dismantling eating as a pleasurable experience to the point where it is effectively loaded not with pleasure but with guilt and association with corporeal 'sin'. We can vividly see in the lives of some young people, including those who speak here, not only the embodiment of damaging, extra-school social forces but some of the problematic, intensified work conditions of contemporary schooling, specifically the commingling of performance and perfection codes (Bernstein, 2000b; Evans and Davies, 2004).

Performance and perfection codes

Our use of the term 'code' is drawn explicitly from the work of Bernstein (2000b: 202), where it refers to the regulative principles which select and integrate relevant meanings (expressed as 'classifications' defining boundaries between people, knowledge forms and objects in time and space), the form of their realisation (expressed as 'framing' or levels of control over the determination of these boundaries) and their evoking contexts (pedagogies, interactions and social relations). The values (strong/weak) and functions (classifications/framings) carry the code potential. How this potential is actualised is a function of the struggle (e.g., between politicians and educationalists) to construct and distribute code modalities which regulate pedagogic relations, communication and context management. Conflict is endemic within and between the arenas in the struggle to dominate modalities and in the relation between local (e.g., family, community) pedagogic and official ones (healthcare agencies, general practice surgeries, schools). In other words, the concepts 'code' and 'modality' (the pedagogical forms they nurture and through which they are refracted) allow us to make connections between macro-trends – for example, in health and education – influences and structures of power and control and micro-processes in schools. They help us trace connections between language, culture and embodied consciousness and indicate how the distribution of power and principles of control in society translate into pedagogic forms and modalities in schools where they are acquired, shape pedagogic consciousness and are 'embodied'.

In previous chapters we have traced the instructional and regulative principles given in obesity discourse whose codes define meanings in relation to people, weight, exercise and food regulation which become embedded in formal and informal school structures so that, for example, even lunchtime practices and playground behaviours that may not at first sight be considered embodiments of the pedagogic device may be of great importance (see Chapter 6). In all cases, pedagogic practices constitute the social contexts through which cultural production and reproduction take place, in which 'difference from', 'similarities to' and 'relations of' the body are realised (Evans and Davies, 2004). Analysing how differing pedagogic 'texts' are put together, decoding 'the rules of their construction, circulation, contextualisation, acquisition and change' (Bernstein, 2000b: 30), becomes the first step in any attempt to understand pedagogic practice and its effects, which is why we indulged in an extended interrogation of obesity discourses in Chapters 2 and 3.

We have approached this question by acknowledging that, in Bernstein's view, two fundamental pedagogic models feature in formal education in the UK and elsewhere. He labels them *competency* and *performance*, each referring to specific procedures for engaging with and constructing the world. Each has a social logic, that is to say an implicit model of communication, interaction and the subject. Each, therefore, expresses a specific set of meanings, systematically reproducing variation in those fields of practice which people inhabit in their daily lives. Bernstein (*ibid.*: 57) discusses both models with reference to the features which they share. Whereas competency modes (CM) focus on procedural commonalities shared within a social class, ethnic or other relevant category, performance modes (PM) focus on something that acquirers do not possess, upon an absence, as a consequence placing emphasis on the text to be acquired and upon its transmission. Whereas CM are predicated on *similar to* relations (what people have in common), PM are based on *different from* relations (what sets them apart). In CM differences are viewed as complementary; in PM as hierarchically distinct. Bernstein stressed that although these models and modes could be considered discretely and gave rise to distinct forms of pedagogy, mixes took place on what he colourfully referred to as a 'pedagogic palette'. Which discourse is appropriated depends on the dominant ideology in the official recontextualising field (ORF), which includes government departments of state and other more specific, often quango-like, agencies, such as curriculum and testing and regulatory and inspectorial bodies and upon the relative autonomy of the pedagogic recontextualising field (PRF), where a range of academic professional, teacher-training and research and commercial agencies, such as publishers, consultants and an increasing army of for-profit and 'philanthropic' venturers (Ball, 2007a) put direction and meaning on official impulse. There was a shift in formal education in the UK from PM to CM in the postwar period up to the 1960s, with a reverse shift from CM to PM from the late 1970s until the present as a result of increasingly direct state intervention in the official recontextualising field, with consequent and, in large part, deliberate weakening and transformation of the PRF from Thatcher's assumption of power in 1979 onwards. Consequently, and despite increased devolution, performance codes and their attendant modalities now define both the culture and the grammar and syntax of pedagogy in the majority of British schools.

If adapted insensitively, Bernstein's characterisation for heuristic purposes of these two contrasting modalities is sometimes allowed to underplay both the presence and significance of other codes whose origins are not encompassed by the social, psychological and behavioural sciences. While Bernstein (2000a, 2001), like virtually all social analysts of his era, gave great weight to the interests of business and industry in his notion of 'production', unlike Durkheim he was not particularly concerned to interrogate how social relations were 'embodied'. The social bases of some powerful influences on pedagogic codes, while not unrelated to the interests of production, lie, as we have argued, in the media, medical and health fields. These focus, among other things, on the dynamic between body and nature and biology and culture, referring to relations of 'the body' rather than relations to or *differences from* individuals and agencies *outwith* 'the self'. In Foucauldian language these refer to 'relations to one's embodied self'. In this respect, they are best characterised as body *perfection codes* which, we suggest, now pervade the cultures and structures of Western societies and are reflected in schools (Evans and Davies, 2004). They represent a shift from a concern with repairing the 'physical body' through specific pedagogical action (for example, through PE and fitness regimes) to protecting/preserving the unfinished body by reconfiguring body, mind and soul through *intervention* and *prevention* as everyone's concern. Indeed, in Chapter 6 we argued that this notion would appear to have a great deal in common with Bernstein's (2001) ideas, where he saw Britain as the emergent 'totally pedagogised society' (TPS), a social order 'shaped, animated and maintained through the discursive principles of pedagogy as embodied in new educational technologies, life long learning policies and a fluid, highly credentialised work force' (Tyler, 2002: 5). Here cognitive and social attributes of actors are to be especially developed in the family, school and leisure for a 'pedagogical future of socially empty trainability' (Bernstein, 2001: 366); 'empty', in Tyler's (2002: 5) view, because it is a 'mere shell for the expansion of consumption, electronic communications and the circulation of the images of global capital culture'. In this context identities are recognised through consumption and displayed through the 'right' embodied capacities, managed by a strong state 'through processes of centralised decentralisation' (Bernstein, 2001: 367). Significantly, the main force of pedagogic relations becomes its invisible, normalising effects through an apparatus of symbolic control which valorises trainability, a capacity for endless forming and reforming of individual desire. The ephemera of unfettered consumer 'choice' serves as surrogate for having any real responsibility or control over decision-making in key aspects of our lives. Such a society depends on its workers' capacity to find meaning not in coherent or stable social relations, commitment or careers, but rather 'in the gratifications of consumerism' (Tyler, 2002: 5). Tyler sees this information-centred modality as another stage beyond its precursors – Bernstein's subject- and student-centred modalities characterised, respectively, as performance and competence. This, then, is the social context in which perfection code modalities are located and emerge, at least in part, as reflections of consumerism and global capitalism's capacity not only to 'manufacture' and manipulate desire and emotion but to define the 'displayable' embodied 'trained' and 'trainable' 'qualities' that, putatively, industry and commerce require and the nation-state needs.

The social bases of perfection codes

The social bases of perfection codes are located in trends outside formal education, as outlined in Chapter 2. Much of their impetus is driven by developments in medicine, epidemiology and healthcare, and the massive proliferation of interest in 'the body' in Western cultures, contexted in an era of 'flexible capitalism'. These are endorsed and supported by the health and media industries in the UK, where it has been estimated that around £1.5 billion a year is now spent on 'gyms', while the health supplements industry is now worth £350 million a year (*Times Magazine*, 2002). These changes have been reflected in obesity discourse and the reorientation of the school curriculum (see Chapter 6). Evidence abounds that teachers and policy-makers in the UK, Australia, the USA and elsewhere are now wrapped in an ideology of 'healthism' orientated, among other things, to making young people more active, 'fit' and thin (Gard and Wright, 2001; Evans, 2003). Within this discourse, individuals are deemed largely responsible for their own health and for 'making healthy choices' as entities relatively independent of structural constraints and cultures (Henriques *et al.*, 1984). Although there are tensions between health discourses and modalities now found in schools, all, in one way or another, focus on the body as *imperfect* (through circumstances of one's class and poverty or self-neglect), *unfinished* and to be ameliorated through physical therapy (circuit training, fitness through sport and a better diet), *threatened* (by the risks of modernity/lifestyles of food, overeating and inactivity) and, therefore, in need of care and being *changed*. Although perfection code modalities share features of performance and competence modalities – and, for this reason, could be seen as 'products' of the pedagogic palette – their dedicated concern with enactment on and regulation of 'the body' leads us to view them as distinctively characterising our emergent TPS, constituting a new, contemporary, Western mode devoted to body-centred concerns, within a wider discourse of embodied capacity for trainability, fitness and health. As we have pointed out, all pedagogical relations are power relations; there is no instruction without regulation, no pedagogy divorced from control. Perfection code modalities are not exceptions to this rule. Indeed, in Chapter 3 we suggested that we might consider the 'ethic' embedded in perfection codes as particularly virulent and explicit, given their enactment directly on body consciousness, determining what bodily acts, shapes and forms are permitted and forbidden, the positive and the negative values of different possible behaviours of, and on, the body. They simultaneously determine and define what 'the body' is and ideally what it ought to be, and provide the ground rules for sifting and sorting those who can from those who cannot either aspire to or achieve appropriate corporeal ideals.

Performance codes and the disordered self

We have also highlighted that perfection codes manifest in obesity discourse are not recontextualised in a social vacuum. They translate to school cultures that are already defined by performance codes and reflected in the intensification of schoolwork, including the increasing pressures wrought by examinations, assessment, expectations for achieving high grades in 'learning' and excelling in sport. These were pressures that had long been more than passing concerns for the young women in our study, as is exemplified by the following focus group extract:

Mia: They're [schools] always talking about what you're going to get in your GCSEs or your A Levels. They never actually really encourage you. They just say, 'Oh, if you don't do that, you're not going to pass your A Levels or your GCSEs,' and then you just worry the whole time.

Karen: I was starved when I took my GCSEs. I wasn't eating and I wasn't drinking. I was sitting there and I couldn't concentrate. I was really dizzy.

Interviewer: Did your teachers know you were ill?

Karen: Yeah, but it was important that I sat the GCSEs and got the grades.

In conversations with both teachers and young women at the centre repeated reference was made to cultures of intensified expectations endemic not just in specific subjects but more generally in schools:

> Well . . . you've got GCSE . . . then they've got AS Level the next year, then A Level the following year and it really is a bit crazy, I think . . . Important exams every year from year 11 is a lot . . . and even the Key Stage 3 exam, which is two years before GCSE . . . although it shouldn't affect the children at all [. . .] the schools make it sound very important to the children: 'You've got to do well in your SATS' . . . and they build up the pressure in a way that perhaps isn't so necessary.
>
> (Mrs Bailey, In)

I think, like, exams make a big stress and, like, peer pressure . . . not about being thin . . . I dunno . . . just about other things and it makes you feel like you can't do that so you've got to do something else.

(Jane, Fg)

I got so stressed out about exams . . . and I just had to control something and then I lost it and I wanted it . . . so badly.

(Vicky, Fg)

Emphasis on competition and ever-rising, never-attainable, perfect academic states was a major concern for Lauren and Carrie, both aged seventeen:

Lauren: What's all this A, B, C business anyway? Why put people into boxes? It just creates competition and resentment.
Carrie: Even if you work really hard and get an A, and then someone else gets an A*, it doesn't matter any more because they have taken it [the achievement] away from you.

(Fg)

These were sources of deep anxiety, where the girls blamed themselves for their failure, their lack of effort in achieving ever-changing, unattainable academic ideals: 'I've been sick again today . . . I'm OK now but I've just been so stressed out recently with essays and coursework . . . I just feel lazy and stupid and that I'm getting worse . . . If I don't get more motivated I will fail and I know I'm going to do really crap' (Claire, Em). Moreover, in their view, the problems they were experiencing not only went unrecognised but were sanctioned and normalised by the performative cultures of their schools and middle-class homes: 'I remember getting so worried and worked up about it. My parents and teachers all just saw it as a competition and didn't really think about how it might be affecting me' (Vicky, In). In such conditions it was hardly surprising that some of these young women classified themselves and were classified by their parents and psychologists as 'perfectionists':

Vicky: I'm a complete perfectionist . . . I have to have control.
Kate: I am at some things but not others . . . I used to be . . . all my books used to be, like, perfect and if I made one mistake I'd rip it out and do my work all over again.
Vicky: So would I.
Kate: Even if it took ages . . . I used to be like that, but since I came here I really don't care.
Jane: I'm not so bad as I used to be . . . I do care, but it's [. . .] not that important any more.

(Fg)

In effect, the expedient, socially constructed conditions of intensified schooling produced by educational policy and practice manifesting performance and perfection codes were routinely interpolated as psychological traits whose damaging consequences were exacerbated as they intersected with other problematic aspects of the young women's lives.

Pursuing 'perfection' through academic performance and meeting cultural expectations, however, often ran directly counter to a desire for recognition and status within informal school peer-group cultures, creating dissonance and extreme anxiety for many. Lauren and Carrie, for example, felt that recognition arising from sporting success was 'good' because it was valued by both staff and students, whereas recognition of academic success was 'bad' because it led to being labelled a 'geek', 'teacher's pet', 'swot' or 'naturally clever'. As Carrie (Fg) pointed out: 'If someone was really good at sport, say at football or something, they were, like, idolised. But if you were good at academic things, then people just took the Mick because you were a swot.' Others, however, reported dissonance between their desire to resist or rebel against convention and the attitudes of peers who adhered to their schools' performative ideals:

> Yeah . . . just like that you had to be, dunno . . . like . . . to be proper and, like, wanting to do well with, like, wanting to be a doctor and stuff or a nurse, or be a lawyer and, like, all the good jobs and that was like everyone wanted to do and everyone was working towards it and everyone was, like, well behaved and no one swore . . . no one did anything wrong, and I just was nothing like that at all . . . I dunno . . . cos . . . I came from exactly the same families as they did. But I just didn't like that.
>
> (Lara, In)

Many of these young people felt that most of their problems at school were 'caused by anxieties about relationships with other people' (Lauren, In). These anxieties, which clearly related to perceptions of what 'people think of you' and 'meeting expectations', connected to a desire either to belong to the 'formal culture' or to one or other of the different peer cultures in the schools or to their endeavour to manage relationships and success in both. Cliques or different friendship groups were, thus, a recurrent theme in the girls' discussions, where various labels were mentioned, including 'popular' (i.e., beautiful/skinny), 'swots', 'sporty' and 'geeks'. It was just a case of 'trying to fit in' (Lauren, In) especially with 'high-status' groups.

Given the pervasiveness of performance and perfection codes in school culture, it was perhaps equally unsurprising that body shape and 'weight', just as James (2000: 29) found with respect to 'height', should be used to 'facilitate the embedding of individual child bodies within the wider social body of school children at school [and] stems from a particular way in which a child's changing physiology is culturally held into account'. Body shape not only 'register[s] the present social status of the child' but 'provides a literal yardstick for a child's status as a future adult'. Effectively, for some, perfection code principles of 'slenderness' become *the* credential for recognition and belonging in a performative culture where talking about and trying diets becomes 'a rite of passage', a means of achieving and displaying what individuals have in common with high-status others in terms of the 'right' body, commitment and attitude. In such contexts, as James (*ibid*.: 28) notes, work on the body is intended to highlight not just the particular body a child or young person *has* but the particular body that person *is* among others. The visceral, emotionally charged pleasure to be derived from visibly pursuing a worthy shared ideal should not be understated when set in contexts where the formal performance code of school routinely differentiates, separates and sets apart these young people. That 'reading bodies' and assessing social relations in such ways were shaped for our respondents by narratives of obesity discourse at the intersection of the corporeal and pedagogic devices was well illustrated by Carrie (Fg), who had learned that 'if someone doesn't like you and they want to pick on you at school, then weight is the thing that they will go for'. Locating 'eating disorders' in these tensions, constraints and pressures that arise in schools and between them and other social spheres, such as family, leisure and work (Holroyd, 2003) is, then, a necessary precursor not just to understanding disordered eating but to seeing it among other forms of 'deviancy', success and failure in schools. All of these young women suggested that schooling played a strong part in the development of their eating disorder, highlighting, to various extents, problematic experiences with competition between individuals for grades, achievement, status, sporting recognition, popularity, bullying, cliques, groups, stereotyping and lack of individual recognition. Their narratives announce the potency of perfection codes in the aetiology of eating disorders and how important it is to set disordered behaviour against the backcloth of intensified schoolwork, a culture dominated and driven by performance modalities and codes.

Perfection codes: social hierarchies of the body in schools

A 'cult of slenderness' is not usually explicitly advocated in formal education, except, perhaps, in specialist ballet schools, elite sports coaching and curricular areas dedicated to body concerns, such as those to which we have already referred (see Chapter 6). It is more often than not transmitted indirectly, albeit in good faith, through the mediation of 'obesity discourse', which has become embedded in school cultures and structures by teachers, pupils and their peers in subtle and incidental ways: 'Look at your hip bones popping out, you're so slim it's unfair' (Claire, Em, reflecting on an exchange between peers). Few young women in our study talked specifically about physical or health education contexts or pedagogies, but all alluded to the raw fear of being placed on 'display' in PE and other 'health' settings:

> and, like, swimming . . . I hate, like, having nothing to wear apart from the costume [. . .] We have to swim with the boys which is really annoying [. . .] and it's even worse if a boy comments on you . . . cos you feel really sensitive.
>
> (Vicky, In)

> Communal showers and that just puts more emphasis on everyone, like, looking at each other [. . .] I think that's terrible [. . .] and then afterwards it

would be all the bitchiness: 'Oh, did you see her or did you see her!' . . . It was terrible.

(Rebekah, In)

They also alluded to the narrow perception of 'health' as a corporeal condition, as an achieved outcome of eating the 'right foods', 'exercising' and achieving the 'right size', reinforced and endorsed elsewhere in schools. These practices and attendant attitudes could be viciously endorsed by peer-group activity and the social hierarchies which some sought to maintain: 'One day in PE we were doing circuit training and in the changing room the coolest girl in our year group came up to me and said I was fat! I was in tears. I lost control. This started some of it off' (Susie, Pd).

Others, like Lauren, Carrie and Ellie, during a conversation about learning about food at school, talked of learning what was 'good' and 'bad', partly through PSHE lessons but also through parents and the media. Jane (In), for example, commented:

At school they teach you about healthy eating . . . like what's good to eat and stuff [. . .] and, like, you get the information . . . they teach you about fruit and stuff and vegetables and bread . . . and that is all, like, good food . . . and, like, chocolate and crisps is bad food, and you shouldn't eat it . . . and I dunno . . . you start thinking about that and you start getting really obsessed.

Among wider socio-cultural pressures, debates about obesity, as presented in newspapers and on TV, were certainly part of Ruth's consciousness when she said: 'They're always going on about obese kids at school . . . the government needs to stop stressing' (Ruth, Em). However, uppermost in the girls' minds were bodily ideals portrayed in the media, which were felt to be inescapably present within other sites of social practice. Lauren (Ic) was clear that she thought these images could, in part, be harmful: 'I'd sometimes like to write to them [magazines] and say, "Do you not realise that you're not being helpful to young people?"' She also commented that when she was ill in hospital, her mum wanted to read to her from some magazines but found this difficult because their content was predominantly about dieting, food, losing weight and skinny role models:

Lauren: You can't look through the pages of something like the *Daily Mail* without coming across 'The Little Black Dress Diet' or something like that.

Ellie: They say things like 'lose weight, feel great, keep it off'. It's always things like that.

Carrie: Yeah, and they always have comments from people who say, 'Oh, it changed my life, I feel like a better person.'

Ellie: And they have 'before' and 'after' pictures of people and they always make them look really horrible beforehand, like miserable and with bad clothes.

Carrie: They use pictures of naturally skinny people all of the time too, so it gives you the impression that if you do what they say that you will end up looking like that and that's not the case.

Lauren: Not only that, but you never see a picture of a well-built teenager in magazines: they're always really skinny . . . I'd love to see someone who had natural beauty, yeah, but also a natural figure.

Carrie: We've been watching [reference to a TV model competition] in here, and we were laughing because all of the people that have got through to the final have got their hip bones sticking out and everything and they were just so bony.

Lauren: But I find that the only reason I have for watching that programme is to try and catch a glimpse of them eating. And there isn't anything.

Carrie: I watch people on TV sometimes. It's quite sad I know, but [laughs] I watch their behaviour and you see the fork going up to their mouth but you never see them eat anything.

Lauren: Yeah, it's like that advert with Kate Moss, when she walks down the road and then she walks through a kitchen, then she picks something up, a strawberry I think, she puts it to her mouth but you don't see her eat it . . . I wonder if they are trying to create the illusion that they are in some way anorexic.

Carrie: Almost like they're perfect and they don't need to eat.

Interviewer: Do you think it's seen as a weakness [to eat]?

Carrie: Oh yeah . . . people have completely lost track of the fact that 'low fat' and 'healthy' are two completely different things. When they advertise low-fat diets they're assuming that they're healthy, and they're not at all.

Lauren: Yeah, I liked everything to be low fat. I doubt if I had one gram of fat a day, but I was aware that I was having five hundred calories and I thought that was enough. I wasn't having fat but I had calories.

Carrie: They make you think that having fat in any form or way is bad, but people then just cut out fat completely. They should advertise more realistically. A diet where you have to inject yourself several times a day and cut out protein can't be healthy. A healthy diet is eating when you're hungry and stopping when you're full.

(Fg)

The upshot of this was disjunction between the expectations of the treatment centre, which endeavoured to address the overemphasis on perfection and performance in both health and academic matters and those reported as 'usual' in these girls' homes and mainstream schools. This created difficulties in returning to school cultures devoid of clear structures for eating and where pressures *not* to eat in order to stay thin were clearly formidable for these girls. These narratives described a 'cultural toxin' that had pervaded many aspects of their homes and schooling. They also revealed the emergence of body hierarchies relating to size, shape and weight (Evans *et al.*, 2002b) induced at the intersection of performance and perfection codes. As Ritenbaugh (1982: 352) pointed out in the USA, the terms 'obesity' and 'overweight' have become 'the biomedical gloss for the moral failings of gluttony and sloth', part of a tendency there, as elsewhere, to 'blame the victim', a culture which nurtures interpretation of fat as an outward sign of neglect of one's corporeal self; a condition considered shameful, dirty or marking irresponsible illness, reproducing and institutionalising value beliefs about the body and citizens. Clearly, when obesity narratives are recontextualised as a discourse of certainty about exercise, food and diet and are taken up within formal and informal school cultures, they may have powerful bearing on individuals' developing senses of well-being and self. As we have seen, especially in Chapter 4, particular body shapes come to be recognised as being of high status and value so that some people become unable to recognise themselves as having bodies and 'selves' of any value at all.

'Hungry to be noticed': achieving self-determination within performative school culture

Schools' perfection and performance codes, mediated by teachers, peers and friends, were interpreted through individuals' powerful desires to achieve recognition of individuality and 'agency' at school which most felt they rarely received. Among them, Mia (In), for example, commented: 'I've found that the teachers in this school, they're very cold and they never talk to you personally, like you're a person. They'll talk to you like you're a number to them and that's all it is basically.' Moreover, Ellie (In) considered that her headmaster 'didn't really seem to care about his students', while Carrie (In) commented that she felt students were not 'treated as individuals' within school but just stereotyped or categorised in relation to ability. Their stories indicated a perceived lack of care about their spiritual, mental and emotional health and development. Consequently, for many, thoughts of returning to 'normal' (mainstream) school evoked a great deal of distress:

Carrie: I've been to several different schools, since I've become ill this is, trying to get away from the illness at school . . . I have actually just been trying to find alternatives to go back to because I know I can't go back to that school for my health, if you know what I mean . . . But in terms of whether school actually started the illness, I really don't know whether it did. All I know was that before I became ill I was immensely, immensely depressed, and I think the depression came from the school.
Interviewer: Because of the environment?
Carrie: Mmm . . . and because I've always been a very insecure person and school provided me with no security whatsoever.

Again, we emphasise that these conditions of schooling do not *cause* eating disorders. However, these girls clearly learn to see food and diet as an acquired 'resource' to cope with the cultural demands placed on them by teachers and peers in these environments. They use their bodies in the power relations played out in schools, with some coming to see anorexia as a horrifying yet desired practice, a resource which, if drawn on over time, becomes deeply sedimented as a habitual way of thinking and acting. Lydia (In), for example, commented:

> There's a lot of bitchiness and of course there's a lot of 'Oh, I look so fat', you know, there's a lot of that going around. You have to look perfect or you're not going to look good, and the popular girls are just going to look at you and go [derisive noise], and you know you don't really want that . . . You don't want to be noticed as the fat person; you want to be noticed as the stunning, skinny person.

In effect, their bodies became outward markers of 'value' in the consumer culture reflected in schools (Featherstone, 1991; Bordo, 1993). The slim body signified 'romantic femininity' associated with a variety of positive psychological characteristics (Wilkinson, 1986) as well as self-control, status and 'worth' (Malson, 1998). For some of these girls it was a way of being heard and of demonstrating self-control, autonomy and individuality and of achieving recognition by peers and others as the end product of disciplined dietary restraint:

Lauren: It's like what I've found at school is that I was just branded, that was just who I was. And I just found that in some cases I could get away with things because I was anorexic and because I wasn't as capable as other people and, I don't know, that was awful really because I want to succeed at life because I'm talented, not because people feel sorry for me.

Interviewer: So it was a label that you didn't want?

Lauren: Mmm, but in some respects I did want it because it made me feel special, it made me feel that I was more important than everybody else, and I think in some ways that was why I couldn't get rid of it at school . . . Because you have 'the dominants', 'the leaders', 'the thinkers'; I was just 'the anorexic', that was who I was. And when this other girl at the school became anorexic, I felt that I had been pushed out of my place and I was furious . . . It [anorexia] shows that you have a strength that others don't, because, let's face it, not many people have the ability to starve themselves to death.

Malson (1998) has noted that some young women quite understandably perceived anorexia as a positive resource, signifying success and control. For middle-class girls like Lauren, self-starvation had come to represent a personal solution to broader social problems, among them lack of order, control, recognition and success within school and her social milieu (see Eckerman, 1997). As Turner (1992: 221) puts it: 'The anorexic avoids the shameful world of eating, while simultaneously achieving personal power and a sense of moral superiority through the emaciated body. Their attempt at disembodiment through negation becomes the symbol of their moral empowerment.' Such comments, however, are rather patronising and fail to capture the ways in which such behaviours are expressions not of a *selfish* but of a *selfless* quest for belonging and recognition in social conditions of schooling and family life that deny some expression of the anorexic's authentic self (see Chapter 8). For Lauren, for example, anorexia is constructed not just as *a* way but as *the* only way of finding a 'voice' and identity which differentiated her from others at school. While her eating disorder might not have started either with such intent or with its realisation in mind, the casting of anorexia and extreme slenderness as positive in terms of achieving some symbolic status and power in school should raise alarm bells about what is inadvertently endorsed by obesity discourse and its many proponents in and outside schools. It seems to lead to at least some young people coming to believe that 'body work' of the sort achieved by Lauren is appropriate if one is to be *valued*.

We need reiterate here, however, that performance codes not only regulate the nature of the health messages relayed in the formal and informal curriculum but define 'health' itself and its 'effects'. In performative culture 'health' has no intrinsic value and no inherent properties, such that these young people have learned that to follow the recommendations of obesity discourse to the extreme is to become seriously ill. 'Health' itself becomes a performance, a process of constant comparison and competition both with one's own embodied self and with those of others, of striving for 'gold standards' with respect to eating and exercise that are themselves volatile, ever changing, never attainable and over which they have little control. The resultant anxieties are inevitable and seem impossible to avoid, as witnessed by Anne (Pd): 'Started cutting down, saw people eating less than me, got worse. Got worried, saw myself getting thinner. Couldn't eat.' Kate's (In) and Tracey's (Pd) respective experiences reflect the invidiousness of it all:

> Yeah, because all the boys used to say, like, how ugly I was and how my best friend was really fit and how I wasn't and how I was fat and she wasn't and how she was really pretty and I wasn't . . . It was really bad.

> Friends, peer pressure, friends not eating, competitiveness against other people, comparing, skinny friends, arguments, friends talking about weight and going on diets, canteen food.

Performative health, thus defined, affords recognition, status, distinction (indeed, some perverse sense of 'well-being') only if it lifts and separates, 'betters' the self in relation to 'others' who do not have the discipline, desire or wherewithal to work on the body. It 'succeeds' irrespective of real costs to physical and psychological 'health'. The achievement of this 'condition' of 'health' is a double-edged sword. Excessive exercise and dieting function to produce an identity that indicates a 'concomitant negative construction of "the self" as otherwise lacking identity' (Malson, 1998: 197), simultaneously signalling not only that one has an anorexic identity but that, without anorexia, one has no identity at all. We emphasise again that the feelings and processes described are not peculiar to 'anorectic girls'. Prout (2000: 5, referring to James, 2000) reported the usualness of how 'material differences in size and weight present children with a series of problems which must be negotiated by working representational transformations that can render them nearer to or further from the bodily appearances of their peers'. These processes are neither arbitrary nor readily endorsed by young people; indeed, some are profoundly antagonistic towards the social hierarchies induced by perfection and performance codes as they experience them in and outside schools:

> I think that less emphasis should be placed on all the healthy eating kind of thing . . . I think everyone should be . . . you know . . . I think there should be more emphasis on how people should be treated the same and not how everyone might look different or might be a different shape . . . and obviously if someone's like clinically obese then you'd need to address it . . . but then that's the same as if you were, like . . . underweight . . . but then I think that should be done privately rather than . . . 'Nobody should eat fat and nobody should eat crisps' and things like that . . . cos I think it's really detrimental.
>
> (Rebekah, In)

The negative effects of obesity discourse and performative culture in terms of tendencies towards surveillance, monitoring and assessment should, in this view, be replaced by a ('competency') culture (and attendant modalities) that sees 'beyond the body' to what individuals have in common, irrespective of size and shape, rather than focusing on what corporeally sets them apart.

Conclusion

Again we emphasise that it is not enough to see wider cultures as 'causal' factors in the development of disordered eating (Lask, 2000). We need to understand how they are transmitted, taken up, learned, endorsed and instantiated within families, schools and other cultural spheres. Cultural stereotypes do play a role in how children and young people experience their bodies, but they do not simply passively absorb them:

> Rather they actively apprehend and use them in experiencing not only their own body, but also its relationship to other bodies and the meanings that were forged from these encounters [. . .] One reason for this is that children have to come to terms not only with their own constantly changing body and those of their peers, but also with the changing institutional contexts within which meaning is given to these changes.
>
> (Prout, 2000: 8)

These contexts are indelibly shaped and formed by performance and perfection codes. Of course, we need further research asking if there is anything about being 'middle class' that contributes towards anorexia nervosa and other forms of disordered eating, while recognising that the aetiology is not class specific. How are contemporary body-centred cultures mediated through structures and cultures of schooling and overlapping peer-group and familial cultures? Global changes in social and economic structures in recent decades have often pushed middle-class females (and males) into uneasy compromises with the self and others. There seems to be a clear coincidence of anorexia and educational achievement, with Bruch (1973: 73) reporting some time ago:

> growing girls can experience [. . .] liberation as a demand and feel that they have to do something outstanding. Many of my patients have expressed the feeling that they are overwhelmed by the vast number of potential opportunities available to them [. . .] and [that] they have been afraid of not choosing correctly.

These processes are mediated through and endorsed by the pedagogical and power relationships that prevail between teachers and pupils and among pupils and peers in schools and other spaces. Admittedly, we have barely begun to address these issues here.

While feminist (Walkerdine, 1990; Blackman, 1996; Skeggs, 1997) and other sociological work suggests that middle-class existence is constituted on the basis of a pathologising and 'othering' of working-class existence, our data press us to reiterate that middle-class girls also 'suffer' through various social and cultural educational processes. The 'hidden price' of middle-class girls' apparently effortless achievements may often be obsessive hard work, guilt and devastating feelings of inadequacy (Walkerdine *et al.*, 2001). This is not to lay the blame for disordered eating and anorexia on teachers and schools, for neither alone are wholly responsible for it. In all of these girls' lives there are many other factors that have contributed to their decisions to embark on, learn and persist with the use of food and self-starvation as sources of comfort and methods of bringing meaning and control to their lives. We are not in a position to do more than indicate these 'other factors', acknowledging that we seek to highlight that the cultures of schooling cannot be ignored as coincident and contributory in the development of these conditions when they should, if anything, be involved in their prevention. Nor do the data presented here point towards simple solutions to eating disorders, for example, in the form of critiques of media imagery. To do so would be to oversimplify both their complexities and relationships with disordered schooling. In the next chapter, we again take up issues of competitive cultures, assessment, performance, heightened achievement and 'academic perfection' that are now so pervasively written into the fabric of schools in the UK and elsewhere. In passing, however, we might note that surveys revealing 'stressed-out seven–eleven-year-olds' and 'pervasive anxieties' among primary schoolchildren about national school tests and many other worries in their lives (*Guardian*, 2007: 1) are a salutary reminder that feeling the 'ill-affects' of performative culture is not the preserve only of middle-class girls and young women in 'high-status' secondary schools.

8   Affective pedagogies

Emotion and desire in learning to become ill

The 'risk' in going to school

In this chapter we set out to illustrate how the pressurised, emotionally charged environments of contemporary education, configured by what we have described previously as 'performance and perfection codes' within a culture of 'performativity' (see Ball, 2004a and b, and below) contribute not only to some of the difficulties that vulnerable young people experience in schools but to the way in which teachers and others respond to them pedagogically and emotionally, often in very 'unhelpful ways'. We go on to suggest that, even if a different, altogether 'nicer', range of emotions is to be fostered, these also need to be handled not just with greater sensitivity, heightened knowledge and different forms of understanding but within pedagogical relationships in which *control* over communication (over the voice of education itself, as well as over whose voice is recognised and heard) is much more evenly shared.

In Bernstein's (2000b: 364; our emphasis) view:

> *The pedagogic relation is that relation which normalises the intimacies of desire, and public aspiration, conduct, and its practices, through its shaping by macro structures.* However, its discourses make available at the level of individual consciousness the means of disturbing such normalisations.

The sociology of education in the UK and elsewhere has been at its best, over many years, when picturing the ways in which formal education 'normalises public aspiration and conduct' through, for example, processes of differentiation, selection, achievement and socialisation in schools. However, at the same time, it has rather neglected other elements of Bernstein's project, not least how the pedagogic relation 'normalises' what he refers to, rather colourfully and playfully, as 'the intimacies of desire', and how these processes occur in and outside schools. It is perhaps unsurprising that so little has been written about this in recent years because it has become, in certain respects, risky terrain. It means dealing with what McWilliam (1996: 306; emphasis in the original) has referred to as the 'erotic' and 'seductive' elements of pedagogic work, the former 'defined in ways that acknowledge its corporeal dimension but *not* a sexually explicit dimension'. In fairness, Bernstein himself did not elaborate much on this element of his project, saying little about embodiment, though his striking phrase usefully reminds us that even the most basic or base aspects of our being, our 'desires' and emotions, are neither arbitrary nor reducible to biology or psychology but are themselves generated, regulated, shaped, worked on and 'normalised' by 'macro-structures', including pedagogic relations, and are therefore implicated in processes of social order, change and control. We have referred to this interplay of the body in culture as an expression of the corporeal device.

With notable exceptions (for example, McWilliam, 1999, 2004; Davis, 2004; Shilling, 2004; Zembylas, 2007), few in the sociology of education have made the affective and embodied dimensions of pedagogy a primary concern. In contrast, psychoanalytic and 'queer' theorists of embodiment have, in recent years, begun to provide rich insight into this dimension of life (e.g., Butler, 1993, 1997; Sykes, 2007). A range of authors working in the sociology of health, physical education and 'the body' has also addressed these issues, often from a Foucaultian, post-structuralist perspective (e.g., Beckett, 2004; Wright and Harwood, 2007; Evans *et al.*, 2004a). Even so, they have not always made direct connection to embodied consciousness and even less so to the subconscious or to how or what individuals teach, learn and 'feel' in schools, or in other contexts in our totally pedagogical society. True, a veritable industry has recently emerged in the fields of counselling and developmental psychology (e.g., Goleman, 2000; Cheniss and Goleman, 2001), around fashionable theories of 'emotional intelligence' (Gardner, 1993) and 'caring' (Noddings, 1992, 2002). This literature has usefully centred attention on the significance of 'emotions' and emotional development among personnel and management in workplaces, including schools. Perhaps reflecting this, curriculum and policy sociologists such as Hargreaves (2003) and Ball (2004a and b) have recently endeavoured to reinstate 'emotions' into analyses of education and treat them as fundamental components of teaching and learning. They, like much of recent work in developmental psychology and counselling, have tended to do so in ways, we suggest, which rather underplay their psychological and sociological origin and complexity and the concomitant difficulties associated with dealing with these embodied aspects of teaching, learning and 'feeling' and 'desire' in schools. Furthermore, in some of the literature where there has been a focus on emotions, it has sometimes seemed to be taken as read that making them a focus of schooling is fundamentally and inherently a 'very good thing'. Research has tended to shy away from exploring not only more negative emotions in schooling, such as alien-ation and disaffection, but the potentially negative uses of emotion in sustaining social hierarchies and effecting social control (McWilliam, 2004; Sachs, 2004). As one of the authors of this chapter once remarked about schools which adopted more personalised, affective, 'emotionally intelligent' forms of management: 'What a lot of emotion you've got on show in your school setting, Headteacher!' 'Yes, all the better to control you with, my dear!'

In his illuminating account of 'teaching and learning in a knowledge society', Hargreaves (2003: xix) argued that: 'teaching beyond the knowledge economy entails developing the values and emotions of young people's character; emphasizing emotional as well as cognitive learning; building commitments to group life and not just short-term teamwork'. He provides an intoxicating agenda that few people, including those pursuing neo-conservative political ones, would want to contest or derail. There is much talk of 'creating environments', 'developing and managing effective teamwork, problem-solving and mutual learning among adults' (and pupils, one assumes), processes that call for a high degree of 'emotional intelligence', not the cold, calculating sort engendered in the 'knowledge economy', but rather the warm, caring, cuddly kind that 'schools with character', as he calls them, in a 'knowledge society' would want to nurture and sustain. These would be schools that recognised teaching as 'not only a cognitive and intellectual practice but also a social and emotional one'. They would be stocked with 'good teachers', who fully understood that 'successful teaching and learning occur when teachers have caring relationships with their pupils and when their pupils are emotionally engaged with their learning' (*ibid.*: 45). While we share these sentiments, they seem, even if only inadvertently, to imply or lead readers to assume that, currently, 'emotions' lie either outside or on the other side of formal education, to be rediscovered, reinstated as legitimate elements of teaching and learning once the knowledge economy is dismantled and the 'knowledge society' prevails.

In the analysis that follows, we take a contrary view in foregrounding how formal education is already deeply emotionally loaded, maybe not with 'the right' or the nice emotions but loaded nevertheless; learning is always and inevitably affectively embodied. In other words, aspects of embodiment and desire are already and always sources of action in pedagogical relationships, whether we register them or not, rather than things 'out there' that need reinstating. This raises the possibility that calling for schools to become more emotionally charged, without some firmer understanding of how emotions are configured and are already at play in educational systems, may be not only premature but not necessarily or inherently a 'very good thing'.

We emphasise here that our interest is not with analysis of the nature of emotions and emotional development *per se* but relationships between affective dimensions of embodied subjectivity and the cultures that prevail in schools. Although, understandably, these issues are often dealt with separately in distinctive strands of the literature, in our view any analysis of emotions – for example, the 'desire' to do well or to 'be distinctive', independent of their constitution through culture and social structure – is likely to provide at best partial and at worst distorted understandings of their content, form and significance in learning and teaching in schools. Something of the complexity of emotions and the dilemmas and challenges of dealing with them was routinely reflected in the comments of participants in our research:

> I'm just all in a mess at the mo [. . .] I just want to do well [. . .] and I'm worried that I won't [. . .] and I know I shouldn't compare myself with other people [. . .] and I know what grades I want to achieve but I feel worried that I won't be able to achieve them! I'm worried that I am just going to be crap.
>
> (Claire, Em)

I'm stressed out. I'm just feeling really unsure and unconfident about my work [. . .] Today I was in an IT lesson and I really didn't like it as I'm behind and I'm useless and I was just welling up listening to the teacher telling us what we have to do, it just made me feel like a failure and I feel like I'm always constantly working.

(Ruth, Em)

If we cannot engage a language of emotion and 'desire' in sociological analysis of education how are we to address these interactions and experiences? The comments of these young women not only highlight the part that schools may play in contributing to serious health problems but offer a salutary reminder that there are no simple, clichéd solutions to dealing with them. Implicitly these young women plead for a different form of schooling which offers less competition, less differentiation and more security, care and support. But, as we will see, they also recognise that even when this is forthcoming, as it presumably would be in 'knowledge society' schools, sympathy without relevant understanding may be no better than receiving no sympathy at all. Their reflections on their anxieties and aspirations reveal troubled identities 'constantly in a state of "becoming" in contexts embedded in power relations, ideology, and culture' (Zembylas, 2003: 213). In such contexts, while teachers may have a degree of control over the nature of the exchanges that take place, some children may feel they have very little or no control at all.

Stephen Ball's (2004a and b) analyses of cultures of professionalism, managerialism and performativity in contemporary education are particularly helpful in understanding affective dimensions of formal education and disordered (not just 'eating disordered') pupil behaviour generally. For our purposes, although his work brilliantly illuminates the impact of these cultures on the subjectivities of teachers, it has little to say about the ways in which pupils, too, are affected by them. Indeed, the narratives of our students allude to this very lacuna. Moreover, Ball has said little about the ways in which these powerful and dominant cultures in contemporary education may intersect with other cultures and codes that find their way into schools via curriculum, classroom and playground pedagogies. These cultures, like some of those described by Ball, have their origin outside the educational establishment in the health, sport or IT industries and are not always immediately apparent in education policy, legislation or administrative strategies, though they can be highly influential in 'determining' the mindsets, pedagogic relations and actions of teachers, pupils and others working within schools and other pedagogic contexts. Ball (2004b: 3) argues that the cultures of 'managerialism' and 'performativity' now pervading formal education have reconfigured the very essence of what it means to be a 'professional', a 'good teacher' and, we add, a 'good pupil'. In this view, the 'pre-reform professional', a teacher 'able to see the value of reflection and the ever present possibility of indecision', has been eroded (if not eradicated) by 'the combined effects of "performativity" and "managerialism"' both of which, Ball suggests, 'perfectly and terrifyingly represent the modernist quest for order, transparency and classification of consciousness prompted and moved by the premonition of inadequacy'. In this view, 'performativity' is

> a technology, a culture and a mode of regulation that employs judgements, comparisons and displays as a means of control, attrition and change. The performance of individuals, subjects or organisations serve as measures of productivity or output, or displays of 'quality', or 'moments' of promotion or inspection.
>
> (*Ibid.*: 4–5)

This cultural manifestation of what we earlier referred to as 'performance codes', along with 'managerialism', 'a device for creating an entrepreneurial competitive culture' (Bernstein, 1996: 75), has more or less dismantled the 'authenticity' of the 'pre-reform professional' and a sense of 'worth' grounded in a feeling of having autonomy, control, responsibility and, critically, the 'trust' of others in 'their' own professionalism. In today's educational workplaces, teachers' effectiveness 'only exists when it is measured and demonstrated and local circumstance only exists as an unacceptable "excuse" for failure to deliver or failure to conform'. 'Post-professionalism' is someone else's professionalism, 'it is not the professionalism of the practitioner'. In effect, in these circumstances, both teachers and pupils experience intensified responsibility without power; obligation without control. Responsibility for their 'performance' refers not to their own judgement as to whether that performance is right or appropriate, but whether it meets others' criteria. They are cultures in which individuals 'have lost their claims to respect except in terms of performance' (Ball, 2004b: 4), not only determining relationships between teachers and pupils and pupils and their peers but, more profoundly, individuals in relation to their corporeal selves. People are defined 'by states of performance and perfection which can never be reached, by the illusion, which always recedes, of an end to change. They are bitter, unforgiving and tireless, and impossible to satisfy' (*ibid.*: 7). Indicatively, we have already noted Carrie (Fg) as saying: 'Even if you work really hard and get an A, and then someone else gets an A*, it doesn't matter any more because they have taken it away from you.' These tendencies are repeatedly reflected in the voices of other young women in our study. For example, Mia (In) recollected:

> It's unnecessary stress, I think so, I really do. But I suppose you can't change that, but just the stress put on this GCSE and A Level thing is so *stupid*, because the only thing that really matters is the A Level thing. The problem is, you know my friend, they always say, 'Oh, GCSEs count and make sure [you] do really well in it' and my friend did *really* well in her GCSEs and she did quite badly in her A Levels, not very bad but . . . and then she went to university and she wanted them to, you know, let her in and she didn't get in because of her A Levels. And, I mean, they say GCSEs are the main things that count but it's not true, it really isn't.

Again, we need to remind ourselves that these cultural tendencies (to paraphrase McWilliam, 1999) are exercised by some *body* on some *body* and that they have profound emotional affect: 'The pressures of doing well in school influenced me to stop eating because I felt it was the only thing I could be in control of. The school needs to focus less on work and more on making sure pupils are happy' (Vicky, Dd). Thus, some pupils, like some teachers, not only become 'spectators' (Stronach and Corbin, 2002: 115) or 'disembedded subjects' (Weir, 1997; Ball, 2004a and b) but increasingly disembodied and depressed in the process. They feel that they have less worth corporeally, less significance, less substance as they lose their sense of 'authentic' self:

> It's just that I like to work hard and that . . . and to like feel in control . . .
> And the fact that I don't feel like that at the moment when I go in makes
> me not want to go . . . I know there's like there's no pressure as I'm not
> doing exams till next year but I still, I still feel pressure about going in, I'm
> a mess.
>
> (Claire, Em)

Ball (2004b: 7) reminds us that new roles and subjectivities are produced in this culture as teachers and pupils 'are re-worked as producers and providers who have to submit to regular appraisal and review of performance comparisons'. Consequently, they may 'feel' that they are valued only for the surface features of their actions and being and for as long as they can perform, 'deliver' and display appropriate behaviour meeting others' criteria. Some 'feel' that they have no use, value, substance or worth beyond a particular subject boundary, school or classroom door, and that they have little or no control over what the pedagogic relation has become or how it should be:

> I got on really well with her [my teacher] and I was one of her favourites.
> I really loved her and then when I moved out of her class she wouldn't talk to
> me any more [. . .] But, like, when you're in their class they love you but when
> you get out they ignore you totally. But I can understand that because they
> shouldn't get emotionally involved. But I've found that teachers in [England]
> were, like, they're very cold and they never talk to you personally like you're
> a person. They'll talk to you like you're a number to them, and that's all it is
> basically.
>
> (Mia, In)

> My chamber choir teacher used to be really friendly until I left her class. Now
> she won't talk to me, she tells me to get out when I go into her room, and if
> I smile at her then she won't smile back. She'll just turn her head and look the
> other way.
>
> (Sophie, Fg)

Here, then, are contexts loaded with emotion displaying, in these girls' perspectives, dispassion, detachment, distance and aloofness, drivers of the 'empty pragmatic self' (Dawson, 1994: 153). As Ball (2004b: 10) contends, performativity bites deeply into our sense of self and self-worth, calling up 'an emotional status dimension, despite the appearance of rationality and objectivity'. Some pupils, like teachers, are 'hurt' in this process, as they are inscribed with value only with reference 'to the diligence with which they attempt to fulfil the new (and sometimes irreconcilable) imperatives of competition and target achievement' (*ibid.*: 9). Yet there is deep irony in this process. As much as these young people resent this culture and its processes they continue to strive to meet its measures of success. As one parent reported:

> Pressure's always a contributor . . . erm . . . I mean, our daughter's a high achiever . . . pretty well everyone you talk to's children are high achievers . . . They develop low self-esteem because they're not satisfied with their performance . . . and . . . they . . . push themselves incredibly hard and are not satisfied. I mean, our daughter got . . . when her GCSE results came through she got nine A*s and an A and she was really . . . pissed off about the A . . . erm . . . and in fact it was a mistake she ended up with ten A*s, but . . . actually that doesn't do them any good, because they then believe that that's a measure of success.
>
> (Mr Ashby, In)

There is, after all, as Ball reminds us, something very 'seductive' about the ways in which 'performativity' is constructed and presented in schools. Those parents, students and teachers who understand the criteria for judgement in this culture and can achieve well in terms of them may feel, at least initially, empowered. As Ball argued, there is always 'the possibility of a triumphant self'. Pupils, like teachers and others in schools, learn in this process that they can become 'more than they were/are'. There is something very seductive about being '"properly passionate" about excellence, about achieving "peak performance"' (*ibid.*: 8). Nevertheless, while all of this involves, in one way or another, 'intensive work on the self' (Dean, 1995: 581), the 'perfection' of such performances is ultimately ephemeral, unobtainable and therefore deeply alienating and damaging to those concerned:

> [This] is what my teachers say: 'You lot have got to stop making all these silly little mistakes! There's a girl in the upper sixth who got top marks, 105 out of 105! She's a very clever girl . . . very clever.' Miss X my teacher said that whilst smiling! Then another teacher said . . . 'It is possible to get full marks, there's a student in upper sixth who's done it! She's ever so clever.' To have teachers say this to you about another student puts so much pressure on us. When they said this I instantly felt I was going to fail, and that I wouldn't ever be clever enough to do as well as she did, especially as she is so clever!
>
> (Claire, Em)

In these circumstances, it is hardly surprising, though rather problematic, that the search for perfection and performance becomes embodied in the lives and personalities of those young people subject to it, often supported and endorsed by the languages of counselling and psychology invoked to 'explain them' which they quickly learn. Some who experience this sense of never being able to obtain what is asked of them in a performative culture gradually define themselves as 'perfectionists' and see only themselves as to blame when they fail. In Mia's (Fg) view: 'because we're all perfectionists, we're all very competitive, we all have the same personality. I think it's a type A in psychology.' These pupils are found in a position of having to 'cope' to protect their fragile educational identities in circumstances that routinely provide opportunities for their evaluation and demise. Pupils who may begin by explaining their failure disparagingly with reference to their teachers are inured to going on more damagingly to complete the explanation with reference to their own ability or embodied selves. If they cannot, do not or will not meet these conditions (the 'currencies of judgement', as Ball (2004b) neatly describes them) then they quickly learn that they have no value, do not fit in and do not belong. Ellie mentioned that her headmaster 'didn't really seem to care about the students, as long as the school achieved', while Carrie commented that she felt they 'weren't treated as individuals within school', but rather just 'stereotyped or categorised' in relation to relevant attributes or abilities (e.g., 'sporty' or 'clever'). 'If you don't fit in to one of the positive categories you can feel isolated and ignored' (Ic) – hence the attention you get from losing weight is welcome. Their stories indicated a lack of care about their broader spiritual, mental and emotional health and development. The important point here is that 'performativity' is 'a struggle over visibility' (Ball, 2004b: 9); individuals, like organisations, mean nothing if their achievements, their presence, cannot be registered and properly 'displayed'. For teachers, for example, this means appraisal meetings, annual reviews and report writing; for pupils, assessment criteria, 'levels of attainment', 'performance indicators' in academic subjects and/or sport. It is an endless, emotionally charged quest for recognition by others, of fitting in, trying to achieve and belong:

> Yeah, well, getting into [my current school] was really pressurising . . . at [my previous school] I was really happy . . . It [my illness] was *all* the new school . . . and I didn't really fit in there . . . cos . . . I'm quite, like, quiet and . . . [my previous school] was, like, a tiny school compared to [my current school] . . . and everyone was just, like . . . I wasn't really there . . . I felt like I wasn't really there.
>
> (Vicky, In)

All this, Ball (2004b) reminds us, occurs in contexts in which there are high degrees of uncertainty and instability and of being judged in different ways by peers, parents and teachers; it is a high-risk enterprise. In such contexts, where the risks of failure are so many and rewards so few, it is hardly surprising that some children take radical steps to ensure that their 'self' is protected, that they achieve some sense of 'belonging' and retain at least a measure of control in their lives.

Losing one's body to become somebody

In these conditions some pupils have problems in thinking of themselves as the kind of 'good' pupil they are 'expected to be', as ones who simply produce 'performances', constantly striving for the academic or expressive 'perfection' that schools, not they, 'need'. Some lose their sense of 'authenticity' because, in their view, the pedagogic relationship is inauthentic, not meaningful and deeply affected as it coldly fails to engage with who they feel they 'really' are. In Ball's (2004b: 13) terms, 'the affective is compromising the effective'. In these circumstances, some individuals feel not only increasingly 'at risk', anxious and insecure, as does Vicky, but 'inessential and insubstantial', and they engage in actions that literally come to embody these attributes. In Jane's (In) words, 'it triggers things when I get stressed over school and I don't really want to eat'.

Of course, once more, none of these conditions 'causes' disordered eating or other disorders of the body but they are, at least in part, contingent 'effects' of the cultures of contemporary schooling. Furthermore, the means of addressing problems experienced in this culture are readily available in the form of 'other' powerful cultures pervading formal education: relating to health, 'obesity' and 'slenderness' (Evans *et al.*, 2004a), and which intersect with and endorse performativity, positioning 'the body' as another form of valued currency in schools. These girls saw self-starvation and their bodies as 'resources' to cope with the 'inauthentic self'. They were 'used' in the power relations which they played out. Their bodies were 'manipulated' to resist the 'inauthentic self', ironically in an effort to regain some sense of moral substance, self-worth and significance in their lives through not eating and controlling relationships with food. Such actions are as intentionally subversive – 'You cannot stop me, you cannot control or regulate who I say I am' – as they are consensual – 'Isn't this [thin, controlled] who you say I should be?' This is an interesting paradox. These interpretations of weight are extrapolated to other aspects of identities, coded into references to accomplishment and hard work. Hayley (In) remarked: 'I always used to look at my friends and think that I wanted to be as good or as pretty or as clever as them. So I decided that not eating was a way that I could maybe achieve that.' In other words, the body becomes just another way of achieving 'performances' to meet the criteria of excellence, control and so on by which they feel they are judged by teachers or their peers. Conversely, it is also a resource for challenging inauthenticity and, in this sense, control over food. The 'expertise' involved in achieving self-starvation may come to represent a personal solution to broader social problems, among them a lack of order, control (Eckerman, 1997) and recognition within schools.

These young women identified thinness as an important goal in the assessment of personal achievement, with their actions endorsed, simplified and legitimised by wider cultural obsessions with obesity and slenderness reflected in central government Policy and school policy initiatives to alter eating and exercise habits, ironically in the interests of 'health'. As we noted earlier, Jane (In) claimed: 'At first it was just healthy eating but I took it to extremes . . . then I started just eating fruit and veg and nothing else . . . and then . . . like the first time I did it, eventually I didn't really eat anything.' Almost identically, Vicky (In) recollected that 'I thought I have to cut down a bit and then I just went to, like, healthy eating over the summer . . . before I went back to [my school] I was always eating, like, five portions of fruit and vegetables first . . . and then at [school] I just didn't eat . . . it all went down completely.'

Many of these girls alluded to a feeling of ontological insecurity within the contemporary cultures of schooling and the paradox of using the body to reassert a sense of self-worth within contexts where the self is rapidly becoming invisible. Through the body the girls intended, once more, to become 'visible'. However, these actions were not mere reflections of that discourse; pedagogic discourses 'make available at the level of individual consciousness the means of disturbing such normalisations' (Bernstein, 2000b: 364). While defining their subjectivity in terms of 'body perfection' these young people also vehemently rejected this version of themselves and of others' bodies. As Vicky (In) claimed:

> I just want my friends to be less stupid about how they do things. It's just like not eating because I have to not eat [. . .] I always felt that the girls got it really wrong . . . and, like, I always felt like everyone around was anorexic too so I had to be as well . . . cos none of my friends ate lunch at school.

They, like Vicky, hoped and believed that they might retain this body form only for as long as it offered status, acceptability, responsibility and the feeling of being 'their own person': 'Well they [peers] would always tell me how, like, . . . skinny I was and they would say, 'Oh, you look so good' . . . Well, one girl said, 'Oh, you look amazing' (Vicky, In). At least, in some fundamental aspects of their lives, they are in control.

Reading the body in a performative culture

Of course, many schools and teachers do engage with the sentiments advocated by Hargreaves (2003) and make efforts to have caring relationships with their pupils. Some of these young women and their parents are able to identify teachers who have, albeit casually or incidentally, provided general sympathy and help: 'they were understanding about it but that's as far as it went' (Mia, In). However, few of them talked positively of the ways in which their schools had addressed their specific concerns or wider health issues: 'They didn't even ask . . . cos I looked quite ill [. . .] but they didn't even ask if everything was all right . . . It was one of the things my mum went into the school and complained about . . . cos they didn't even . . . Nothing . . . not a thing' (Rebekah, In). Within a culture of performativity, while efforts are sometimes made to engage emotionally with, to have 'sympathy' for, such young people, teachers often do not have the time or the knowledge, or the discursive resources to read beyond the surface features of their behaviours. Instead, they focus on individuals as sources of 'display/performance' and as body/weight concerns, which compounds students' problems of getting significant others to see 'beyond the body' to who they 'really are'. Lauren (In) commented:

> One of my teachers came up to me and said, 'Oh, how have things been?' and I said, 'Oh, not too well. I think they're thinking of putting me back in a unit', and he goes, 'Well, you don't look too thin' and I was like [sighs], 'But you don't understand, there is more to it than just being thin' ... And also when I came back to the sixth form, the same teacher saw me in a corridor and the first thing he said to me was, 'Are you putting on weight?' He shouted it across the whole corridor. He saw me and it obviously triggered in his head, 'Oh, weight issue, are you putting on weight?' and I was like 'Oh my God!'

It is not only the content, the messages relayed, but the form of relationship and exchange that matters here – in Bernstein's terms 'their classification and frame', the boundaries and hierarchies that are defined between teacher and taught and the levels of control each 'enjoys' in the encounter. Lauren, unsurprisingly, was clearly uncomfortable with this exchange as it drew attention to the surface features of 'her' disorder and, significantly, she had little or no control over how she was being 'read' and 'displayed' in these contexts. It was an instance of pedagogical power relationships over which she had very little influence. Our point, however, is that it is unsurprising that the body is read in this manner. As many have pointed out (e.g., Bruch, 1973; McSween, 1993; Peterson and Bunton, 1997; Evans *et al.*, 2004a), in Western cultures of performativity and corporeal perfection, where 'the body' is constantly subject to authoritative gaze, health educators, teachers, doctors and others simply assume rights of judgement over the 'other's' body and its health, with their actions sanctioned by the authority of obesity discourse. In the process, relationships between the private and public are sometimes cruelly dissolved, without the approval of the 'object of the gaze'; in this case, Lauren. Hayley (In) recalled a similar interaction when her mother had made her have lunch with her sister, who was in a higher year group, 'which was bad enough'. Then, 'One time a teacher had made a comment when I was in the lunch queue at school. She said, "Well, Hayley, is this really you in a queue for food?" It was awful. I mean, especially there in front of all those people.'

Disordered eating, indeed any disordered behaviours, are extremely complex and difficult conditions for anyone to deal with, including 'trained' health professionals. Again, we do not wish to lay blame here, but rather to highlight that even when efforts are made to engage with the more emotive features of pupils' lives via demonstration of sympathy, comfort, encouragement and support none may in themselves be 'good' or 'productive' features of pedagogy if not accompanied by understanding and mutual control over communication and exchange. In the cases above, the less the girls became corporeally, the more they hoped that others around them would see them for who they 'really were' and recognise the difficulties they experienced within and beyond school. Ultimately, however, within a culture of performativity, the focus became the surface, bodily features of weight and size, rather than understanding of their educational, social and emotional struggles. In Jane's (Ic) terms: 'They [teachers] think it's all about, like, food and weight, so if you put some weight on then you're better . . . Yeah . . . cos . . . the weight is just the trigger of it . . . it's not the cause.' Carrie (In) also commented that teachers 'didn't seem to understand just how much was going on in my head. They thought, I don't know, that I was being stupid or trying to get attention or something.' Meanwhile, Mia (In) recalled similar feelings and experiences:

> Mmm, not just what happens, because that was what I was taught, and not just what happens physically but what happens mentally. People don't often realise what extreme pain and agony it is. They just think it's like a glamorisation of getting attention and things like that. Which is not true.

The 'desire' to lose yet more weight and do more exercise in a vain endeavour to achieve recognition derived its meaning from the conditions of schoolwork and its perceived, increasingly distant, unattainable goals. It makes no sense to consider such feeling or desires as irrational expressions of maladjusted or absent psychological traits. We therefore reiterate that emotional empathy without altered understandings or changes in the nature and content of the communication of pedagogic authority and control, despite the best intentions of schools and teachers, is likely to be inimical to the well-being and interests of young women, such as Vicky (In): 'And they've [teachers] got all these stereotypes, like . . . in the science book it was . . . erm . . . "these eating disorders are when you choose not to eat and you get painfully thin", and it's just, like . . . it's nothing to do with that at all [. . .] It's so much more . . . it makes people sound really shallow.' Whether the 'pedagogies of desire' advocated by others (McWilliam, 1996; Zembylas, 2007) would provide the possibilities for teachers and students to press beyond such tendencies, to question such normalising representations of the pedagogic body so as to 'reconfigure it . . . as corporeal and relational, yet undetermined and unambiguous' (McWilliam, 1999: 218, quoted in Zembylas, 2007: 341), is an issue requiring further investigation.

Caring cultures?

Where do young people – such as Claire (Pd), who took the view that 'Teachers don't understand. [There is] no one to talk to that understands' – receive the attention they require when schools, peers and, in some cases, even guardians or parents endorse the cultures of performativity and body perfection that they are so eager to avoid? Clearly some of the young people quoted above felt that they lacked control. There was much they wanted to say to reinstate and to value themselves, yet alarmingly, like Lydia (In), they felt unable to voice these concerns either in school or with their families:

> All I can do is try and talk to them [parents and teachers] about it, but, you know, 'The issue is here, Lydia. You know you've got to get better,' and I'm, like, 'Shut up.' And you know they don't really want to know what I think, because they're like, 'Why can't you eat?' and I'm like, 'Why can't you understand?' It's really, really frustrating.

Schools were rarely considered places where their problems could be voiced. On the contrary, they were, as already mentioned, deemed part of the problem, as Lauren's (In) comments that were noted earlier remind us: 'All I know is that before I became ill I was immensely depressed, immensely depressed, and I think the depression came from school.' Perhaps unsurprisingly, some of these young women suggested that it was only through unique relationships formed with other young women or adults, often outside school, who were suffering from or had experienced an eating disorder that they could construct the narratives they wanted to relate to others about their embodied identities, sense of worth and problematic relations in schooling. Counsellors, carers and teachers inside schools were considered less than helpful if they could not 'share' the experience of disordered eating, or if they read such behaviour reductively, concentrating only on its surface features: eating and weight. Vicky (In) recollected:

> I think there should be people to talk to about it so they know, and so that your parents . . . there should be, like, a counsellor or someone but . . . the thing is with a counsellor is, like . . . I would prefer to speak to someone who's had the illness and has got better . . . and not just a counsellor.

Of course, the turbulence of adolescence – filled, for some, with struggles, confusion, secrecy and shame about the body – may lead us to question how much information teenage girls and boys are willing to disclose comfortably to adults in any context. For those young people who do feel disempowered in schools and, sometimes, even among their peers, we might wonder where, within a culture of performativity and corporeal perfection, they can express these feelings of disaffection and alienation. Evidence elsewhere is beginning to suggest that this perhaps partly explains why the internet has emerged as a key medium for the expression of such narratives (see, e.g., Walstrom, 2000), allowing young people to feel that, at least in this pedagogic relationship, they, rather than adults, have a greater degree of control.

The forms of 'radicalism', via control of food and their bodies, that these young women engage with, then, are not generated counter-intuitively by the pedagogic relations of formal education, or at least not exclusively so. There is little evidence of class counter-culture or inversion of school values here. These girls 'resist' conventional cultures and structures of schooling which are deemed to be uncaring and indifferent to their complex concerns by simultaneously reproducing elements of performative culture, on the surface displaying a very 'middle-class' desire to be and stay thin, while consciously rejecting it by taking this endeavour to 'unacceptable' extremes. In this form of resistance centred on the body and diet, constructed via and sanctioned by more 'global knowledges' within obesity discourse about health and the body and formed through recontextualising agencies, such as the media and the internet, they at least feel they have some sense of control over how their bodies, identities and selves might be read. As far as they are concerned, there are few if any locations in school to where they might escape to avoid the routinely damaging effects of performative cultures, despite the efforts sometimes shown by some staff to show some concern.

Teaching and learning in a knowledge society

McWilliam (2004) has implored researchers to ask critical questions of the rediscovery of 'emotionality' in educational administration and leadership. She has asked why emotions are being evoked for educational leaders now, how it is being done and what its effects on educational leadership and management are likely to be. In this chapter we have tried to illustrate that emotions, while undoubtedly personal and private, are inextricably related to public issues, cultures and macro-structures; and, critically, to questions of authority and control. We have been inclined to view the emotions expressed by these young women as akin to the 'productive desire' to which Deleuze and Guattari (1987) refer. For them, desires were neither defined as a *drive* in a Freudian sense, nor as a *lack* in the Lacanian psychoanalytical approach (Zembylas, 2007). On the contrary, they proposed that desire, as a 'material entity', always has a socio-political context: 'There is no such thing as the social production of reality on the one hand and a desiring production that is mere fantasy on the other . . . *There is only desire and the social and nothing else*' (quoted in Zembylas, 2007: 335; emphasis in the original). In this view, for Zembylas (*ibid.*: 337), desire

> is an assemblage of heterogeneous elements; it is a process, not a fixed structure; it is affect, as opposed to feeling; it is event, as opposed to thing or person. Desire also implies the constitution of a field of imminence or a body without organs, which is only defined by zones of intensity, multiplicity and flux.

We share this view, while noting its tendencies ultimately to dissolve the significant presence of a physical body in time and place, the interplay of biology and culture, or what we have referred to as the meeting of the corporeal and pedagogic devices. Notwithstanding such limitation, this view of 'emotion' does imply that 'if social meanings and ideologies are constituted in power relations and desire relations, then it is necessary to look at social institutions (e.g., schools) in terms of their networks of power and circuits of desire' (*ibid.*: 336). It also entails asking, among other things: 'what are the conditions for new ways of living and desiring?' (*ibid.*). The emotions expressed by the young women in our study must be viewed in this light as relational and as irreducibly contingent 'effects'. Their descriptions of school cultures alluded too often to 'inauthentic' experiences in schools wherein they felt devalued, with little sense of individual identity, self-worth or control. Their 'desire' to alter their sense of well-being, to reshape themselves, had no meaning outside the institutional structures and interactions which had produced such feelings in the first place. For them, the critical issue was not how they were to receive and experience greater 'emotionality' in the pedagogy of formal education but how the pressures of performativity and corporeal perfection could be coped with and how the right to participate, speak and be heard for 'who they were' and 'how they felt' in pedagogical processes could be achieved.

Finally, we return briefly to Hargreaves' (2003) inspiring book to look again at the detail of what might be involved in creating the 'schools with character' and the 'teaching with heightened emotional understanding' that he advocated. One is reminded here of Bernstein's (1971) injunction that in organisations where relations are weakly classified and framed, where pedagogic relationships between teacher and taught, knower and known, knowledge and learner are more 'integrated', flexible, fluid and 'open' (as they would be in 'knowledge society' schools, one assumes), more, not less, of individuals' emotional, social and physical states becomes open for surveillance and potential control. Beyond advocating obvious structural changes in formal education, we also need to ask what knowledge(s) or what alternative educational codes (what ethics and ontologies) are to be enacted in these contexts if students are to feel valued, and from where are they likely to emerge? Whose and which knowledge(s) will legitimately prevail?

'Curriculum supplements' in the form of media literacy programmes addressing, for example, representations of the body, slenderness and heath are an insufficient means of addressing such aspects of the cultures of schooling that are so damaging to some students' and teachers' health. Creating 'schools of character', it seems to us will require radical changes not only in the structures of schooling (for example, in the relationships between teacher and taught) but in the cultures, ideologies and contents of education that will give rise to less differentiating ways of speaking and thinking about individuals and health. This will include an onslaught on 'performativity', some clearer understanding of what its cultures are to be replaced by, and greater appreciation of the discursive representations generated in recontextualising fields, such as the media and information technology, outside education that increasingly inform teachers', pupils' and others' understandings of what it is to be an embodied learner. Knowing how and where learning is to occur, not only in schools, will require a new body pedagogic eschewing performance and perfection ideals. If nothing else, the voices of the young people in our study remind us repeatedly that appeals for more caring, affective forms of schooling, unless accompanied by some substantive, critical understanding of the knowledge(s) that should inform such processes, may mean little more to students than schooling loaded with sympathy and goodwill which, if lacking relevant understanding, action or alteration in power relations, may be worse than receiving no sympathy at all.

9 Alternative pedagogies
Rethinking health

Alternative perspectives on health and weight

As we have progressed through our analyses the voices of young people have vividly revealed the potentially damaging consequences of obesity discourse, especially when uncritically recontextualised by teachers and others in and outside schools. They remind us that pedagogy, in relation to the body, exercise and weight, is not just about 'content', particular messages and belief systems prevailing locally, nationally or globally but entails a set of relationships affording teachers and pupils different levels and forms of responsibility and control. We have heard young women lament being 'invisible', 'ignored' and powerless in a performative school culture, impotent to change their circumstances, despite being constantly on display, monitored, assessed, compared and judged. Some are so overwhelmed by constant pressures to be successful in meeting the expectations of parents and schools that they simply 'give up': 'it is strange because sometimes I feel like I don't care' (Vicky, In). Claire (Em) attempted to explain why this happens:

> A lot of teachers forget to praise and just state the crap parts . . . making students feel incompetent and unable to do exams. The fact students feel 'dumb' will have a negative effect, as students will be less likely to put effort into revising, as they will see no point as they believe they will have already failed! Also when you start to believe the negative thoughts you will start presenting the thoughts through your actions, i.e., if you feel like you can't do something then you won't be able to do it.

All had used their bodies as resources either to distance themselves from or to resist this culture, announcing the alienation of their 'authentic self' from society and school. Jane (Pd), for example, succinctly encapsulated the problematic relationships between performative culture, obesity discourse and her devastating ill health: 'Exams, depression, self-hatred, happiness gone, ugly, fat.' She, like others, pleaded for less judgemental, more reflective and humane forms of education and health to that traded in their schools' performative culture which granted them greater responsibility and control.

For such reasons, in this chapter we want to examine some perspectives offered in recent theoretical work on health and obesity which resonate with these wishes and provide alternative ways to begin to rethink health and construct alternative pedagogies within society and schools. In so doing, we offer conceptual tools for 'reading' obesity and alternative discourses critically, while underlining the importance of grounding health practices and initiatives in the material, socio-economic and cultural circumstances of people's lives. We do this by turning to a variety of perspectives which currently lie submerged beneath dominant discourses within nutrition, physiology, epidemiology, health science and medicine that offer alternative, more cautious and circumspect readings of 'weight' and 'health' than is evident in much 'mainstream' obesity literature. We suggest that unless policy-makers and educationalists embrace some of these alternative perspectives and acknowledge the social class, gender and other socio-cultural and economic conditions that influence people's choices and opportunities to be healthy, their analyses of health behaviour are unlikely to create either policies or pedagogies that have a lasting and positive impact on people's lives. When 400,000 children and young people reject celebrity chef Jamie Oliver's version of what is good for them in respect of what they should eat for school meals, reflection is called for about disjuncture between the aspirations and interests of working people, the desires and maturational needs of their children and worthy but dislocated/ disconnected middle-class ideals (Clark, 2007: 4).

Many of the alternative perspectives that we draw upon in this chapter are concerned with 're-evaluating the weight-centred approach toward health' (Cogan, 1999: 229). Collectively, they help us rethink constructions of 'health' and obesity and associated health policies in more complex, humane and democratic ways. A number of these perspectives take what might be termed a humanistic approach to weight and fat, challenging their cultural stigmatisation as harbingers of size/fat acceptance. While groups, such as the US-based National Association to Advance Fat Acceptance, have become advocates of changing negative socio-cultural and medical attitudes towards fatness, others are more concerned to critique the scientific validity of claims underpinning obesity discourse. As outlined in Chapters 2 and 3, a range of studies now provides evidence which challenges some of the core assumptions and claims of obesity discourse and its medicalising tendencies. These perspectives argue that 'dominant interpretations of obesity . . . are based on incomplete and imprecise information' (*ibid.*). For example, a growing body of research has demonstrated that overweight is not directly associated with excess mortality (Flegal *et al.*, 2005) and that being 'overweight' does not preclude health or well-being. Gregg *et al.* (2005) report that obese people in the USA have better cardiovascular disease risk profiles than their leaner counterparts of twenty to thirty years ago. This body of work suggests that weight outside of the extremes may not be the issue at all in terms of health-related risks; to focus on 'fatness' as a social ill in this way is to invoke size discrimination and might be characterised as a form of 'civilised oppression' (Rogge and Greenwald, 2004, cited in Aphramor, 2005: 332). Such dissenting voices within obesity discourse may help nurture more complex understandings of socio-political and physiological aspects of 'fatness' if given the authority to do so. This would require a 'power shift between competing groups operating with separate conceptions of health, away from biomedicine and towards more socially rooted understanding' (Duncan, 2004: 177). However, as Monaghan (2005b) has observed, the obesity debate is hardly a debate at all and these alternative perspectives often occupy a marginal position in obesity discourse. Indeed, 'size acceptance' movements and studies that draw upon critical social theory to make sense of 'the obesity epidemic' are not only marginalised but demonised for distracting attention away from the more serious issue of finding medical cures and preventions for ill health. In such discourse one is positioned either on the side of righteousness (the business of making more people thin) or against it, negatively labelled and criticised for obstructing this enterprise and eroding its incontrovertible virtues and underlying truths. There is no in between. Not only are particular versions of health rendered obsolete, but ways of researching it are diminished in this process. As Lupton (1995: 1) observed over a decade ago:

> Due to its close links with biomedicine, which favours positivistic forms of inquiry based on the gathering of quantifiable data, public health research has tended to undervalue more humanistic, critical and theoretical and interpretive approaches [which] have been marginalised; at best treated with suspicion, at worst denigrated for being 'soft' and 'non-practical'. The tendency has been to accept the prevailing orthodoxies of public health and promotion, focusing on statistical measures, cost effectiveness and the evaluation of measurable effects, but devoting comparatively little attention to the critical analysis of the political implications of such endeavours.

Again, we point out (see Chapter 6) that legitimate expertise is constructed within an ethical discourse. This discourse is constructed as 'truth' and 'certainty', while ambiguities and uncertainties within the science itself are seldom made visible in the public domain. For example, representatives of the British Medical Association have advocated that obese children should be taken into care; healthcare must be rationed and priorities set, implying that a particular set of moral decisions have to be made (Miah, 2005). Obesity scientists have become moral commentators on their own science, their views sanctified by what they deem to be children's best interests. While most, we suspect, would find it objectionable were ethicists or social scientists to step outside their realm of expertise in making such judgements, medical expertise has ostensibly become impervious to critique. Overreliance on scientific or medical engagement with ethical issues to fill in gaps relating to cultural and socio-economic realities in matters relating to obesity has meant that public health promotion has tended to be addressed through a language of individualism and moral panic.

The dangers and unintended consequences of currently dominant forms of obesity discourse have been revealed in a great deal of research that has drawn attention to the increasing incidence of disordered relationships with food and the body and underweight among young people. However, such evidence has not achieved the same standing or status in current political discourse, and the research and development funding associated with the approaches to obesity that are currently privileged. It is disarmed by the moral overtones of such dialogue and the narrowing of governments' health agendas in schools towards managing weight, implying dedication to making people exercise and eat less rather than achieving healthy weight at any size or shape. Consequently, as Austin (1999: 246) points out: 'failing to consider the intersection of food, bodies, and diet in its cultural complexity [gives] scientific credibility to our society's obsession with dieting and loathing of fat and is implicated in the promotion of a cultural climate that generates eating disorders such as bulimia and anorexia nervosa.' Like many others to have emerged in the sociology of health and cultural and feminist studies in recent years, Austin's views call for broader ethical and moral discussion about obesity, such as may generate more meaningful public engagement.

Offering alternative narratives might not only assist those who are labelled 'overweight' to reposition themselves but might contribute to wider political, social and cultural discussion on how we are to make sense of obesity. As Gard and Wright (2001: 537) have pointed out: 'media coverage of "expert" knowledge produced in reports serves to generate a public/popular discourse which speaks to politicians and funding bodies about the levels of community concern generated around the issue and so motivates further discussion'. On this basis, alternative discourses may, in turn, enhance the possibility of shifting focus away from weight loss as a central feature of health in relation to public policy discussions on obesity. Unless the moral dimensions of obesity discourse are made public, educators, parents and health professionals will continue to be ill equipped to adopt more cautious attitudes towards the ways in which weight and health issues are normally represented. Failing this, there will be little space for those who are both over-weight and healthy to have visible and legitimate cultural space. To create these alternative spaces, we need to ask different questions about cultural representations of obesity and their legitimation in a variety of social contexts and associated pedagogical fields.

The politics of health: a politics of pedagogy

Is it possible to achieve a form of pedagogy 'with a central focus on redefining success away from the current focus on weight loss, towards promoting a healthy lifestyle, long-term amelioration of medical problems and improved quality of life?' (O'Dea, 2004: 263). Schools, after all, are disciplinary institutions (Foucault, 1980) drawing on contemporary discourses and various normalising techniques in the social construction of young people's bodies and the regulation of their lives. This link between wider, contemporary discourses and schooling processes is particularly relevant to our discussion because 'popular culture is so significant in doing pedagogical work on the body' (Tinning, 2004: 227). Addressing these wider processes, therefore, requires not just a politics of health but a politics of pedagogy, since schools are now positioned as key institutions in the fight against obesity. This requires engagement in a politics of how 'we' (teachers, teacher educators, health workers and researchers) are to construct the experience of education for young people in a way that does not alienate them by separating 'body' from 'mind', 'subject' from 'object', or individuals from the communities and cultures to which they belong. It also requires a politics *of* and *for* the creation of schoolwork conditions that will leave children and young people feeling they have both a stake in the processes and outcomes of learning and, critically, some degree of control over them. Much of the data reported in this book implore us to ask whether current, uncritical allegiance to existing health education priorities is more or less likely to help children and young people achieve these things. Does it leave them feeling confident, competent, comfortable with and in control of their bodies, able to participate intelligently in decisions about food and health as well as the range of physical cultures that potentially feature in their lives? (Evans *et al.*, 2004). Are they equipped with the physical competences to do so and critically knowledgeable of how those opportunities may be framed and constrained by the many vested interests that define their relationships with their bodies and physical cultures? Or, as our data suggest, does it merely leave them feeling that they have no say in such matters or that they are to blame if they do not achieve these things? To suggest that we build a curriculum on the underlying assumption that children and adults are to blame if they get obese or self-starve, become sick and die is one of the most pernicious aspects of contemporary health trends. It is particularly hideous when applied to children and young people and to reduce aspirations for education, including PE or health education (HE), to the triumvirate of 'fitness, exercise and food'. To ask to be judged on these matters alone is to pursue not only illusory but dangerous ideals. Indeed, once those who cost and pay for education discover that the PE and health professions cannot and never will be able to achieve them, they may begin to consider the subject matter of PE and the content of health initiatives to be expensive luxuries, unnecessary rather than indispensable accessories in the curriculum. In effect, fitness, exercise and diet may be in danger of becoming, if they have not already become so, in some quarters the PE and HE Emperor's new clothes (Evans *et al.*, 2004b).

Whose expertise matters?

Should expertise lie with 'education' or with making children active, fit and thin? We share Gard's (2004a: 69) view that, if nothing else, claims of 'special expertise' demand of those involved with educating the body, as in PE and HE, a more critical attitude to issues of overweight and obesity: 'a passive orientation towards scientific knowledge would seem at least out of step with contemporary discussion about the need for *students* in universities to exercise a critical judgement when evaluating the knowledge claims of others'. Many of the young women in our study advocated a similar point of view. This does not constitute an attack on well-meaning pedagogues or researchers currently endeavouring to throw light on children's health and well-being but rails against the way in which research evidence is simplified, evacuated of social and political nuance and contingency and, therefore, distorted as it is recycled for public consumption in the form of official reports, academic texts and, thereafter, school curricula (see Chapter 3). Science, at its best, does not offer certainties, and we should be on our guard against those who, for whatever reason, lay claim to having found them. Professional health educators, teachers and teacher educators need to be vigilant, constantly seeking 'truth' as best we know it, sceptical of the assertions, ideologies and opinions that pass for knowledge and certainty in the official obesity field. The latter have come to supplant a decent philosophical rationale for the teaching of PE and HE in and outside schools. As we have noted, in the UK, as elsewhere, schools are increasingly under pressure to embrace greater responsibilities for the health education of children and young people – they are now replete with health initiatives. For example, since 2002, schools in England and Wales are obliged, as a 'new' National Curriculum requirement, to promote 'personal, social and health education and citizenship' across the curriculum. At the same time, powerful agencies outside schools, influential in the development of school sport, are, with reference to rising 'obesity levels', pressurising PE to place health on the agenda of the sports colleges now flourishing in England (YST, 2002: 7). Every Child Matters and the Healthy Schools Programme (see Chapter 5) are further examples of the many and varied measures now being taken to address these concerns.

Much of this could be good news. Children, properly *educated*, could leave schools not only with profound and critical understanding of their unique health needs but also of ways in which these have been constructed, manipulated and, perhaps, obfuscated by the interests of the 'health industry'. The data presented here, however, suggest that HE and PE, reduced to and driven by the unreflective rhetoric of 'obesity discourse', are likely to privilege curricula, teaching and learning in which success and achievement are defined not in terms of knowledge, understanding and competence but body shape, size and weight. New, invidious social and ability hierarchies are tending to emerge in PE and other HE settings, atop which reside not those high on cognitive perspective but the 'able' and willing to get active, fit and thin (Evans *et al.*, 2002b; Evans *et al.*, 2004a). This is not what young people need or deserve. No matter how well configured, or how much time they are given in schools, PE and HE are no more likely to make children fit, eat well and stay or become thin than is maths to make them multi-millionaires, although teachers in these subject areas may want their pupils to leave school sufficiently numerate and physically literate to become both of these things, should they so choose.

Critical health perspectives

According to O'Dea (2004: 260), although 'weight control is only one aspect of overall child health, it appears to be the dominating current perspective within health education and health promotion initiatives aimed at children and adolescents'. Myriad school-based obesity-prevention and physical-activity initiatives are now in place, though few, if any, conclusions can be drawn as to their efficacy (see Davidson, 2007). Indeed, as O'Dea (2004: 260) insists, 'preventative activities must be examined for their unintended negative outcomes such as those known to result from unsupervised weight control attempts among children and adolescents including growth failure'. While recognising and enjoining the need for such awareness, the practical question facing us is how we might begin to incorporate alternative perspectives that define health more broadly than merely weight, size or shape, especially if teachers are currently obligated to fulfil policy requirements which define health as an 'accountable' and 'measurable' feature of school practice. In the UK, for example, the Ofsted (2005) framework for school inspections now requires inspectors to look at schools' contribution to children's health and well-being, as well as their academic achievement. In such policy contexts, as we pointed out in Chapter 6, it is very difficult for teachers and pupils to resist performative health requirements. Given this, rather than aiming to remove anti-obesity strategies, some responses have become more concerned with simply developing ways of implementing official strategies more sensitively and safely. For example, there are a number of education programmes, including some in media literacy, that provide various conceptual tools for young people to read obesity discourse critically. For Cogan (1999: 229), collectively these programmes presage a more fundamental 'paradigm change that reflects a more comprehensive approach towards the promotion of good health'. In terms of school policies and practices this involves development of a health education that underlines the importance of grounding practices and initiatives in the material circumstances of people's lives, giving young people 'voice' in PE, health and sport contexts and searching across disciplines to establish alternative understandings and conceptions of 'health'. We outline some of their lineaments below.

'Do no harm' within current frameworks?

> Before Governments and other agencies leap into actions that they assume to be beneficial in the battle against child obesity, we must remember to employ one of the most important principles of modern medicine and prevention science, 'First, do no harm.'
>
> (O'Dea, 2004: 259)

Teachers are confronted on a daily basis with a particular orientation towards the body, health and weight within both official and informal policy texts and are under considerable pressure to meet the requirements of anti-obesity programmes. The first perspective we explore acknowledges that anti-obesity strategies are likely to be ever-present features of school policy and practice which teachers are obliged to implement and should find ways to realise safely. Physical educators and health educators, in particular, are seen as being able directly to 'influence lifelong attitudes toward physical activity through their roles in schools and the community, and play a critical part in the prevention and treatment of obesity and/or associated health consequences' (O'Brien *et al.*, 2007: 308). Within a culture of performative health, much of what teachers are required to undertake in schools by way of weight management measures is carried out with good intentions, sanctioned and normalised with reference to government Policy. Yet, over many years, in

Tinning's (2004: 219) view, 'notwithstanding what we know as a result of our theorising and research about how certain cultural practices contribute to limited, restricted or oppressive bodily practices, we have seen little significant systemic changes in such practices'.

However, schools are now also being targeted as implementation sites of eating disorder awareness programmes, though not with the same level of public awareness, political endorsement or equivalent government funding as in the case of weight management. Teachers and health educators are now faced with the difficult task of 'normalizing body image and eating behaviour among a large proportion of our young population' (O'Dea, 2004: 259), while also having to implement anti-obesity strategies in schools. O'Dea argues that teachers' roles in this process are therefore complicated because of the concerns that we must 'do no harm' in our efforts to ameliorate both issues in schools. This 'do no harm' perspective is arguably one of the most realistic and achievable alternatives available, given teachers' obligations to pursue official policy goals. It emphasises that they should at least be equipped with awareness that, despite their best intentions, they may inadvertently be doing more harm than good. Yet, as O'Dea (*ibid.*: 260) recognises: 'the unintentional creation of body image and weight concerns, dieting, disordered eating and eating disorders is a probable outcome of child obesity prevention programmes that focus on the "problem" of overweight and refer to issues of weight control'. Moreover, as Aphramor (2005) and Cogan (1999) observe, seldom are the health risks associated with weight fluctuation made public. Ironically, a culture which has turned the pleasure of food into a guilt-laden eating ordeal may be doing a great deal of damage to the health and well-being of young people, their identities and sense of self-worth. Pathologising food in this way can lead to young people having no pleasurable relationship either with it or with the people, parents, guardians and school-dinner personnel who provide it. Given the rapid rise of disordered eating, it seems imperative that cultivating a critical attitude towards obesity discourse should form a feature of health education in schools, where, if children are to be warned of the risks of obesity, they must also be properly educated on the dangers of weight fluctuation and weight loss. Yet, in Russell-Mayhew's (2006: 254) view:

> Although eating disorders and obesity are related, too often they are seen as having competing agendas. Efforts to prevent obesity are seen as dangerous in promoting precursors to eating disorders (O'Dea, 2005) and efforts to prevent eating disorders are seen as encouraging complacency about healthy weight . . . [D]espite recommendations from leaders in both fields about the advantages of integrating prevention of eating disorders and obesity, little has been done to bridge the gaps between the two fields.
>
> (Neumark-Sztainer, 2005)

The 'do no harm' criterion attempts to integrate both these perspectives while implementing anti-obesity strategies and at the same time, raising awareness of the dangers of disordered eating practices. Encouragingly, 'School-based programmes targeting eating disorders are being developed, along with guidelines (Connolly and Corbett, 1990; Ransley, 1998) and curriculum material (Ikeda and Naworski, 1992)' (Dixey *et al.*, 2001: 216). While issues of bullying, self-esteem and body image may be dealt with in several areas of the curriculum and policy guidelines for schools, there is an obvious need to link these with nutrition education and to ensure that HE messages about the importance of maintaining healthy body weight do not adversely affect those who are larger or fatter than average (see Dixey *et al.*, 2001). None of these measures will be deemed either adequate or meaningful, however, unless they engage students in dialogue and register how their lived experience of class and culture can be represented in pedagogical processes.

Alternative health programmes

Other perspectives driven by humanistic education ideologies or alternative belief systems (Shilling, 2007) attempt to work more fundamentally towards what might be described as a paradigm shift in education and health cultures involving development of more holistic approaches to health. Given a performance-saturated culture, one might be left wondering, however, where there are spaces for change to be found in the interplay between body knowledge, education and physical culture (Evans *et al.*, 2004a) to develop such alternative curricular and pedagogic approaches to nurturing health, weight and the body. What extant or less than moribund belief systems may we call upon, or reprieve, to achieve such ends? Advocates of fundamental shifts in thinking about health call on pedagogues and policy-makers to consider how schooling might be reconfigured to meet both individual and community education and health needs in ways that reflect 'competency' rather than 'perfection' codes. The former centre attention on what children and young people have in common, building on their existing virtues, values and predispositions and enhancing their well-being rather than focusing on what sets them apart or what ideally they should become (Evans and Davies, 2004). This would incorporate a social critique of concepts concerned with health, obesity and the body that enabled students to clarify their personal values and those of others and teachers to gain better pedagogic understanding of the social contexts within which physical education themes have emerged and developed conceptually. For example, a number of school-based HE and critical pedagogy programmes have attempted either to counter the claims of obesity discourse or, more specifically, to improve young people's body image and embodied identities. Various programmes of this sort take different philosophical and pedagogical approaches to health. Recent work by O'Dea (2007) entitled *Everybody's Different* offers guidance on implementing a positive approach to teaching about health, puberty, body image, nutrition, self-esteem and obesity prevention that allows teachers to develop a 'body-sensitive classroom'. O'Dea (2005) had earlier provided a comprehensive review of programmes and major issues surrounding preventative interventions for body image, obesity and eating disorders in schools, while also outlining self-esteem and media-literacy approaches that have produced positive results in some large, randomised and controlled interventions. For example, Smolak *et al.*'s (1998) programme based on earlier work by Smolak and Levine (1994) positively affected children's perceptions of fat people but not eating patterns or weight reduction attempts, nor their propensity to tease fat children. The enduring efficacy of such programmes and their effect on body consciousness are very difficult to assess. They may be a necessary but not sufficient condition for changing attitudes and behaviour, especially when they do not reach out to wider institutional structures or embrace community, peer-group and familial values.

A variety of media-literacy programmes have also now been designed to enhance young people's critical awareness of the stereotypical imagery of the body found in popular culture. Many of these programmes have produced limited results. K. Oliver's (2001: 161) research and development work with adolescent girls in the USA, for example, highlighted the limitations and difficulties of engaging with critical media tasks: 'despite the pedagogical possibilities of using images from popular culture to engage adolescent girls in critically studying the body, there were also many other attendant struggles involved in this type of curriculum work'. These struggles included the need for wider political, institutional and social change, alongside the task of encouraging greater individual reflectivity and attitudinal change. Furthermore, our research, like Hepworth's (1999), highlights that media-literacy programmes rarely address fully the complexity of the relationships between culturally induced images of the body and eating practices, or those between young women, men and other elements of their lives, including the performative culture of schools.

Attempts to engage with more democratic pedagogies that assist young people in resisting contemporary imagery about the body are, however, not always straightforward or easy to implement, especially if, as some suggest, schools 'are moving further from models of, or spaces for, "effective democracy" in which young people can be active participants' (Tinning, 2004: 219). Other perspectives are therefore grounded in critical pedagogies that draw upon the sort of approach which Wright *et al.* (2006: 716) describe succinctly: 'if young people are to recognise how truths are constituted it behoves those who seek to educate them to provide the means by which they have choices in the discourses they take up and to understand the effects of their positions on themselves and others'. For example, in New Zealand, a socio-ecological perspective has been adopted within the health and physical education curriculum which encourages students to understand health not through the language of individualism or performativity but as grounded in the material, social and cultural circumstances of their lives (see Burrows and Wright, 2004b). This is particularly significant in the current 'blame the victim' climate induced by obesity discourse, since healthy choices are no longer reduced to an individual's responsibilities but, instead, are seen as intimately connected to the wider socio-cultural milieu. Moreover, well-being is viewed as encompassing not just biological aspects of health but physical, social, mental, emotional and spiritual features of a person's life. Such approaches may, for example, allow young people to explore how 'health can be achieved by overweight people without dieting and weight loss' (Jonas, 2002: 47), for whom 'self-esteem', not 'fat', may be a primary concern. Indeed, there is a strong case to be made for weight loss to be abandoned as a goal for those who are considered overweight or obese in favour of focusing on other features of health. For example, Ikeda *et al.* (2005: 203) believe that 'promoting calorie-restricted dieting for the purpose of weight loss is misleading and futile. We advocate the adoption of a health-at-every-size (HAES) approach to weight management, focusing on the achievement and maintenance of lifestyle changes that improve metabolic indicators of health.'

Good health is not defined by body size or shape but is a state of physical, mental and social well-being. Shifting teachers' ideological beliefs to incorporate these perspectives is not easy, given that:

> Physical educators, and particularly those more socialized in the PE envi-ronment, display a strong negative prejudice toward obese individuals that is greater than that displayed by other groups. These prejudices appear to be supported by an over-investment in physical attributes, and ideological beliefs.
>
> (O'Brien *et al.*, 2007: 308)

This approach advocates the pedagogising of hybridity in PE teacher education programmes towards an acceptance of the multiple, transgressive and diverse physicalities that young people bring to schooling.

Finally, the role of teachers and other health professionals in the prevention of disordered eating and eating disorders should not be underestimated. As Zembylas (2007: 343) has noted, 'a pedagogical approach which recognises that learning discourses and performances are not absolutely determining can begin to provide teachers and students with spaces for reconstructing their relations'. In this view the possibilities for action include the creation of pedagogic relations that nurture and advance new, inspiring, culturally sensitive pedagogies. And although Zembylas reminds us that we may not be able to prescribe strategies that can help teachers and pupils (and parents and guardians) avoid normalisation 'because it is all too well known that even radical trajectories often become systematised' (*ibid.*), those outlined by Piran (2004: 1) may have particular salience for our critique of obesity discourse and weightism in schools, suggesting that if teachers (and, we add, other health professionals) are to engage in more constructive interactions between themselves and students in areas related to the body, their training should include at least three key components:

> informing and raising consciousness about central issues related to the experience of the body; focus groups and experiential exercises that invite teachers [and all other health educators] to examine and constructively utilize the impact of their own past body-anchored experiences on their current behaviours as teachers [or health professionals]; and collaborative brain storming about possible teachers' initiatives in integrating this knowledge into their own classrooms and into their schools.

Furthermore, like Piran (*ibid*.: 4), we would also highlight that teachers and all other health professionals can work towards such goals of countering pervasive social prejudices about people of heavier weight and body fat only 'if they assume a critical perspective towards adverse weight related misconceptions and prejudices' and their framing in obesity discourse. We share such ideals and, with Piran, would argue that the long-term goal surely must be to create shifts that will allow teachers and all other health professionals to work not only against transmitting weightist prejudices to students but, even more proactively, to counteracting such prejudice. In achieving this, professionals dedicated to the education, health and well-being of all young people, rather than just their weight management, may ultimately arrive at a situation of 'Being (Rather than "Doing") Prevention' (*ibid*.: 1). In the absence of politicians and educationalists willing to engage with the ethics, corporeal consequences and social relations of performative culture, we will remain some way from achieving the ideal of Every Child Matters, irrespective of their size, weight, shape or contribution to a school's academic ideals.

10 Health education, weight management or social control?

The four fat fabrications of obesity discourse

We began this project with modest aspirations, simply wanting to understand better the lived experiences of children and young people. In particular we were concerned with relationships, if any, between their expressed 'private troubles' in relation to their bodies' size, shape and weight and contemporary 'public issues'. The latter has been noisily framed in popular discourse as a global rising tide of obesity, a primary antecedent of ill health. As parents, educationalists and researchers working in body-centred trades (PE, sport and health), we found ourselves increasingly in contact with students and children who seemed to be ever more dissatisfied with their bodies. Some were so deeply disaffected as to be taking drastic, even dangerous, action in relation to exercise and weight loss. We were concerned as to the potential saturation of popular culture by images celebrating slenderness and alarmed at the way in which contemporary discourse about obesity seemed to be normalising and making a virtue of the slender body morph. There seemed to be little investigation of, or dialogue between, medical discourses of 'overweight' and 'underweight' and little documented, critical reflection within the health community on prevailing orthodoxies. Given these circumstances, we set out to investigate currently dominant assertions of bioscience about health discourse and to explore their refractions in popular culture and school policies and pedagogies. If nothing more, we hoped to illuminate processes by which young people learned about their bodies and health and whether current health discourse had anything to do with their body disaffection or problematic relationships with exercise and food.

Fabrication 1: There is a crisis (for health, science or truth)

We set out first to deconstruct current bioscientific wisdom, investigating core beliefs and assumptions about the antecedents and consequences of 'obesity' and 'overweight', appraising the knowledge that now passes for the orthodoxy which we referred to as 'sacred health knowledge' in public and personal discourse on health. We found much wanting. Belying the authoritative confidence of the claims being made in this field, the more we searched for knowledge certainty backed by research evidence that would legitimise contemporary emphasis on weight loss, exercise and fat, the less we found. If there was a crisis it seemed to lie more with bioscience's reluctance either to demur from or debunk its own core assumptions and ideals or reflect explicitly on the morality of its practices and strategies than with population weight gain and associated 'ill health'. The ambiguities, contradictions and uncertainties that riddled the knowledge base of the primary research field (see Gard and Wright, 2005) pointed to the first fabrication now embedded in the policies and practices of schools – *that there is an obesity crisis to be found*. Given that science is designed not to tell lies, Ball's (2006: 153) reminder is timely: 'fabrications' are not untruths but 'half truths or nearly truths', 'simply' offering versions of reality which do not exist, in this case with respect to persons and their health. They are not 'outside the truth but then neither do they render simply true or direct accounts – they are produced purposefully in order "to be accountable" [. . .] Truthfulness is not the point – the point is their effectiveness.' They characterise both the health 'market', where there is serious competition for scarce financial resources, and schools, where teachers have to meet the expectations of inspection and appraisal regimes. They work on and in organisations, persons and populations to achieve 'their transformational and disciplinary impact . . . To be audited, an organisation [or person] must actively transform itself into an auditable commodity' (Shore and Wright, 1999: 570, quoted in Ball, 2006: 152). Their existence impels us to ask a different set of questions of contemporary health discourse concerning its purposes and pedagogical 'effects'. If crises had been simply 'storied into existence', what purposes did they serve? What was it that had to be solved? Following Bernstein's theoretical insights, we sought to interrogate contemporary health discourse's inherent instructional and regulative principles and components in order to register both the forms of communication and the embodied relationships these might engender and their effects upon young people in communities and schools. We acknowledged that while deconstructing obesity discourse exposed its inherent principles and regulative (social/ethical) and instructional codes, this could not be at the expense of dissolving its core categories, such as potentially 'erases experiences that are produced by these very terms in the daily lives and social networks of many people' (Warin *et al.*, 2008: 2), including those of children and young people in schools.

Fabrication 2: The crisis has to be solved

One of the seemingly irrefutable core assumptions of obesity discourse is that there is a crisis which has to be solved, preferably by early intervention in parenting and the school curriculum. Much medical and health policy expertise is now devoted to this end. However, our investigation of the social and ethical encoding of obesity discourse leads us at least to consider that the mantra 'this crisis must be solved' is perhaps the biggest fabrication of them all. New forms of governance depend on continuous crises, entailing creating and fabricating problematic social conditions in which the state can 'reasonably' intervene. The exercise of biopower on behalf of individuals or populations unwilling or incapable of regulating their own or their offspring's behaviour who pose a risk to both their own and others' health constitutes such a case. Without crises and risk there can be no grounds for intervention, testing, weight-loss or health-promotion strategies, norm setting, no effective means of achieving social order and population control. Indeed, in the absence of such measures more repressive state power, unpalatable in a democracy, would necessarily pertain. What Ball (2007b: 18, citing Foucault, 1979: 170) observed in his analysis of recent education policy in general as the state exercising both biopower (in the management of the health and diet of the bodies of the population) and its moral guardianship (in the disciplining of unsatisfactory parents through 'a whole set of instruments, techniques, procedures, levels of application, targets') encompasses what we have reported here, especially in our analysis of health policy in totally pedagogised society schools. However, it was never our intention to provide a detailed narrative on the social origins or purposes of public health discourse through either a socio-historical analysis of obesity or a class and cultural analysis of its current form, important though both would be to establishing the character of their regulative codes. We have been primarily concerned with the more limited objective of understanding how obesity discourse, produced and rationalised in the biosciences, was mediated through the interplay of contemporary popular culture, education policy and pedagogy and, thereafter, recontextualised through the actions of teachers and young people in schools. But if there was no health crisis, what needed to be solved? What social purposes did its fabrication serve? What social and ethical, as well as 'health', codes were being fostered in this discourse and with what effects on education/health policy and ultimately on young people's understanding of their own and others' health?

We alluded, albeit briefly, to the child-saving crusades of the nineteenth and early twentieth centuries to highlight how the medicalisation of social policy served certain socio-political purposes and to sanction ever more intrusive and ubiquitous control over working-class people's lives. Then, as now, crusaders were driven by far more than concern for children's ill health: they were also seen to be addressing the risks posed by inadequate or irresponsible working-class behaviour to the wider social order. Health messages traded moral and social as well as health/ medical codes in establishing new norms around a range of 'correct' behaviours. Such crusades, like those of the eighteenth century, were not only focused on the misuse of food. Borsay (2007) observed how other cultural malaises of this period such as binge drinking, street anarchy, parental neglect and a government in denial (all familiar tropes of contemporary political and media discourse) would have been familiar to mid-eighteenth-century London cultural commentators, as illustrated by Hogarth's painting of 'Gin Lane'. Media-constructed panics characterised both periods and symbolised not only their obvious signifiers or tropes such as overdrinking or overeating but wider anxieties about social breakdown and disorder. In the eighteenth century, as now, 'problem drinking' was one of many behaviours described as out of control and illustrative of a broken society in media-driven moral panics, where reforming campaigners played leading roles in elevating problems to crisis status. In the contemporary context, health agencies, government spokespeople and popular experts take on such reform roles. Borsay believes poor diet and 'binge drinking' do not merit comparison across these periods; of more interest are the moral panics fuelled by pressure groups and the media, amid perceptions of government complacency, that characterised them. Of particular significance is that in all these periods women's behaviour and family breakdown are focuses of attention. As Borsay observed, the women portrayed in 'Gin Lane' are not eighteeenth-century 'ladettes' but wives and mothers seen to be sacrificing their children's welfare to Mother Gin. Problem drinking, like the problem feeding or eating with which we have been concerned, is depicted as both a public and an urban phenomenon. But whereas in the eighteenth century young people were depicted as the victims of their binge-drinking parents' neglect, today their own binge drinking is the main focus for concern, with UK public Policy flailing around without obvious success for ways to make our drinking habits 'more French' by extending licensing hours. In contrast, in contemporary discourse over problem eating, both parents (if working class or single parent) and children tend to be blamed.

The similarities between earlier and current moral panics concerning binge drinking or the misuse of food are striking. They become disturbing when encoded in policy texts and school social relations that have bearing on the lives of young people as they categorise and stigmatise some of them for holding the 'wrong' (while privileging others with the 'right') attitudes and predispositions. In Australia Warin *et al.* (2008: 12) have pointed out that even when the macro-environment, health-promotion focus[1] is targeted at very young children, young people and their families, 'it is women (as primary schoolteachers and childcare workers) and particularly mothers who are the forefront of such strategies . . . as they are the household and community members who are most actively engaged in and organising the day-to-day nutrition and activities of young children'. However, these strategies do not impact upon all women in the same way, for people's daily lives are shaped not only by gender but by social class. As Warin *et al.* (*ibid.*) point out, class-based aspects of habitus, such as employment, have powerful bearing on understanding of and decisions about food. In their study they found working-class women shocked to think that they might be called obese, something at odds with their own experiences of body size and weight. They recounted experiences of food insecurity, poverty and neglect that profoundly affected the ways in which food and nurturing featured in their own families. Low priority assigned to weight loss was not only related to their gender but to differing class habitus. Middle- and upper-class women did not recount biographies of food insecurity but lifestyles in which attention to the body was much more salient, with constant discussion of the need to modify it through dietary and exercise regimes, such as trying a range of diets or attending diet and other groups including gyms. With similar tendencies evident in the UK, it is hardly surprising that the middle-class young women in our study refracted such ideals, defining 'health' as the desire to be, or display, being thin as not only a moral responsibility but a social virtue and, at least initially, something of a personal crusade. If regulation and disciplining of populations and individuals rather than amelioration of their 'health' is the under-lying or accompanying, unintended goal of obesity discourse, the intense pressures and anxieties experienced by young people are unlikely to dissipate and their seemingly 'private', though publicly induced, 'health problems' will neither recede nor disappear.

Fabrication 3: Your health, your responsibility; only you are to blame (and shame)

There is another fabrication critically related to the above. It insists that individuals rather than other antecedent or contingent socio-economic or environmental factors are the primary resource for the resolution of health problems and associated risks. Albeit unintentionally at times, P/policy texts and pedagogies can foster a culture of shame and blame in schools which can contribute towards disaffection and ill health. The idea is endemic in media reporting and implicit in P/policy texts that health problems are essentially the fault of individuals, especially females, or the ignorant, or poor, misguided working class. This is perhaps the most invidious feature of obesity discourse. It distracts attention from the complexity of health issues and specific social and economic conditions, over which people may have little or no control, that structure and set limits to their lives. Indeed, in passing, one might note the following commentary by Routledge (2007: 31) on information released in the UK by the Office of National Statistics:

> The great Victorian statesman Benjamin Disraeli coined the term 'Two nations' to describe a Britain he saw as cruelly divided between rich and poor. That was in 1845. But you could still say the same thing today. Despite 10 years of Labour Government, the UK is still split between a healthier richer south and a less healthy impoverished north. In the dockside Middlehaven area of Middlesbrough, healthy life expectancy – the age people can expect to reach before ill health sets in – is 54.9 years. In the Ladygrove neighbourhood of Didcot, Oxfordshire, people can expect healthy lives until they reach 86 – more than three decades longer. The other social indicators tell the same story of divided Britain. In Middlehaven, only 29 per cent of adults are in work. Didcot boasts 86 per cent. Up north, 27 per cent are owner occupiers. Down south, 66 per cent. Car ownership – 94 per cent for the richer folk, and 29 per cent for the poorer people. These figures are taken from the first detailed survey of the north–south divide carried out by the Office of National Statistics. The report makes grim reading. Nine out of the worst districts for early onset of ill health are in northern cities. And nine out of 10 places with the longest healthy lives are in the south. Disraeli spoke of two nations 'between whom there is no intercourse or sympathy, who are as ignorant of each other's habits, thoughts and feelings, as if they are dwellers in different zones, or inhabitants of different planets'. More than 160 years later, these nations-within-a-nation do live in different places. And they might as well be on different planets.

As we have argued elsewhere (Evans and Davies, 2007), social class is not simply a discursive artefact, a category, or a construction of either governments' or academics' classificatory schemes. It is a visceral reality, constituted by a set of affectively loaded, social and economic relationships that are likely to influence strongly, if not determine and dominate, people's lives. These involve dynamic processes within and across many social sites or fields of practice (Bourdieu, 1986), particularly in families and schools. These are not just contexts in which orientations to the body are nurtured, expressed, some rejected, others assimilated, affirmed and endorsed but locations of opportunity and cost where physical and intellectual capital is distributed and legitimated, and sometimes withheld. In the UK, maybe even more than elsewhere, class has long guided our views of 'others' as of more or less value and has led us to pass judgement on their food, drink, clothes, houses, shapes and the way they treat their children and even their pets. Yet, for all its impact on our daily lives and even though it exhibits continuous change and reformation, it has become something of a forbidden research area, somewhat overtaken by others in the officially privileged, conceptual fashion parade. It just does not seem to cross or even surface as an explanatory category in some people's minds, even when inscribed as a body shape that we are expected not to want.

With Warin *et al.* (2008: 11), we would suggest that a 'gendered and class analysis of health issues and obesity discourse provides a different entry point for examining "obesiogenic environments" (Egger and Swinburn, 1997) by pointing to how social meanings and practices [around health] are embedded and reproduced in everyday lives', including those of middle- and working-class young people in communities and schools. Indeed, without a better understanding of the way in which class, gender and ethnicity are culturally inscribed in educational and health practices, we are unlikely to set meaningful and realistic agendas for either research or policy and practice in schools. Like Warin *et al.* (*ibid.*: 1), we are concerned both to understand and enhance the health of populations and individuals by 'problematis[ing] the universality of health promotion messages and highlight[ing] the integral role that a critical theory of "habitus" [or "lived experience" and the "corporeal device"] has in understanding the embodiment of obesity' and various forms of resistance to it. Again, we would emphasise that understanding how people's lives are shaped by gender, culture and their social class would constitute a vital element in the 'alternative' strategies outlined in Chapter 9. We are under no illusion as to the serious limitations of our data where there are notable lacunae in the narrative, particularly with respect to the voices of males, working-class females and ethnic diversity. Yet, if we are to stand any chance of explaining why some of the behaviours and exchanges relating to health occurring in formal learning are so lacking in meaning to certain sections of the population (for example, some working-class boys, their parents and ethnic fractions), we first need to understand what is meaningful to those individuals about their own participation among peers in school and community contexts, particularly in relation to their understandings of their bodies and health. Moreover, again like Warin *et al.* (*ibid.*: 11), who argue that 'popular discourses continue to privilege and validate the slender female body', we too would emphasise that even where there is a focus on 'gender' in popular culture and academic literature, it is often simply equated with girls or women, despite a 'growing literature that examines relationships between men and their bodies [highlighting] some clear differences in their gendered consumption and embodiment of food and shape' (see, for example, Monaghan, 2005a and b, 2006a and b). Given an approach which 'pathologises and stigmatises fatness' (Carryer, 2001: 90) [. . .] 'the rich diversity of female shapes, the association of the body with women's sexuality and the natural increase of weight with age has been rendered inherently problematic' (Carryer, 1997: 107) (quoted in Warin *et al.*, 2008: 11). A clear message emerges. We are unlikely to appreciate or understand the nature and development of corporeal disorders, or, more broadly, the aversions young people develop for certain aspects of education, including those designed to enhance involvement in physical activity and health, unless we embrace class, gender and ethnicity (Azzarito and Solmon, 2006; Azzarrito, 2008) in both our analyses and the strategies we devise to resolve these things. In their absence, all talk of refocusing attention away from individuals and towards 'obesiogenic environments' and of 'bold whole system approaches' to obesity involving 'partnership between governments, science, business and civil society' (Foresight, 2007: 2) will seem like froth on the surface of politics and an obfuscation of people's real-life socio-economic difficulties and everyday pressing concerns.

Fabrication 4: Fabrications of the self and corrosions of the soul: an outward display of compliance to performative ideals

The voices of the young people in this study repeatedly allude to how the values of individualisation refracted in school P/policy and pedagogy contain the elements of a 'new ethics', based essentially on the principle of 'duty to oneself' to eat properly, exercise more, lose weight and look after your own health. As others have noted this completely contradicts another, traditional view of ethics in which 'duties are necessarily social in character and adjust the individual to the whole':

> The new value orientations are thus often seen as an expression of egoism and narcissism. But this is to misunderstand the essence of what is new about them: namely, their focus on self-enlightenment and self-liberation as an active process to be accomplished in their own lives, including the search for new social ties in family, workplace and politics.
>
> (Beck and Beck-Gernsheim, 2006: 149)

Such processes have predictable effects, as in an individualized society

> inequalities by no means disappear . . . They merely become redefined in terms of an *individualization of social risks*. The result is that social problems are increasingly perceived in terms of psychological dispositions: as personal inadequacies, guilt feelings, anxieties, conflicts, and neuroses. There emerges, paradoxically, a new immediacy of individual and society: a direct relation

between crisis and sickness. Social crises appear as individual crises, which are no longer (or only very indirectly) perceived in terms of their rootedness in the social realm. This is one of the explanations for the current revival of interest in psychology. Individual achievement orientations similarly gain in importance. It can now be predicted that the full range of problems associated with the achievement society and its tendencies toward (pseudo) legitimations of social inequalities will emerge in the future.

(Ibid.: 150; emphasis in original)

Many of these tendencies were pedagogically embedded and embodied in the actions and attitudes of the young people in our study. Their lives had been badly affected by the 'individualisation of social risks' that had been refracted in their school curriculum and pedagogy and written into their subjectivities by contemporary discourse about health risks and the pursuit of slender ideals. They had become experts at managing risks, such as of getting fat, not fitting in or not doing well, while following the recommendations of performative culture to be measurably thin via managing food intake, taking exercise and achieving weight loss to the extreme. As we set about exploring their insights into contemporary health-risk culture and how and why they had taken such radical decisions in relation to their bodies and health, nothing could have prepared us for the richness of their viewpoints and their depth of feeling, their rage and desire to express their opinions over a range of issues, particularly their previous experiences of 'health education' at school. Although often classified by professional 'others' as 'dangerously ill' and therefore, as voices that should be considered either limited or flawed, it was evident that these were not disordered, discordant or deviant voices but thoughtful, incisive, critical perspectives on their lived experiences over a variety of terrain. Necessarily, they were often couched in language given to them by their doctors, counsellors and therapists. To be sure, 'people understand themselves as selves through the stories they tell and the stories they feel part of (MacIntyre, 1984)' (Frank, 2006: 434) and these young women often spoke through the narratives of psychology or therapy with which they were more than familiar. Such narratives sometimes blamed them or their genetic make-up ('perfectionist by nature') for the problems in their lives in ways that were unhelpful if allowed to undermine the authority of their voice or obstruct exploration of the multiple factors that they identified as underlying the trajectory of their radical weight loss, in context, over time. It was evident that multiple conditions, mediated through popular culture and school pedagogies, had deeply affected the life experiences of these young people and nurtured body disaffection, propelling some towards serious eating disorders. Even cursory conversations with them suggested that, among myriad factors influencing their relationships to food and their rational decisions to lose weight, schools featured prominently, sometimes decisively so, in dismantling their pleasurable relationships with both exercise and eating. These relationships, invariably mediated by popular peer-group culture, were profoundly antagonistic to what they felt were their 'real' or 'authentic' selves, who they wanted to be. In the perspectives of these young people their 'radical', dangerous approach towards food and exercise had been normalised in obesity discourse and ubiquitous school health practices which were seen as contexts in which unhealthiness had become a virtue, dieting an ideal, presaging an endless quest for health perfection signified in being, or becoming, thin. These were not 'causal connections' between education and eating disorders but, rather, complex contingencies in which the corrosive effects of performative health culture, in combination with other problematic elements of young people's lives, nurtured and rationalised 'disordered' behaviour. Therein lay the makings of the fourth fabrication, of the self, involving an outward display of compliance to performative culture while inwardly loathing its ideals.

Giddens (1991: 91) contends that where there is an 'existential separation' from the 'moral resources necessary to live a full and satisfying existence', a situation he sees as endemic in late modernity, individuals may experience personal emptiness and alienation. In the context of this study we have seen that in the search for authenticity and meaning in a performative culture some young women, by virtue of their class location and values, seem to be inescapably placed in an endless search for authenticity and recognition beyond their capacity to meet performative criteria of either academic or health success. They seek 'visibility' and 'recognition' for who they 'really' are among peers and teachers in a culture that nurtures neither of these things. In effect, they embodied the 'dark side' of the corporate project and performative culture in their apparent complicity to its ideals, in their own ways 'drawing attention to the subjugation and totalitarian implications of its excellence/quality prescriptions' (Wilmott, 1993: 515). The fabrication we talk of here, then, is of the 'apparently' compliant self, as individuals (the young women) come to terms with the contradictory demands of being one's 'real' self, more than a 'body', in a performative culture which reduces them to a commodity while meeting the expectations heaped on them by families and schools. This was a particularly serious problem for middle-class girls.

Such fabrications are, as Ball (2006) has also observed, of necessity usually based on a limited range of representations or versions of the person or organisation. These versions are written into existence by performative education and health texts and involve the use and reuse of the right signifiers: for example, eating the right food, doing the right amounts of exercise, being the correct shape, while enthusiastically pursing academic ideals. They offer versions of the person (or an organisation) which may not exist but are still produced purposefully in order 'to be accountable'. As already mentioned, *pace* Ball, 'truthfulness is not the point' – the point is their effectiveness both in informal and formal appraisals by peers and adults in and outside schools; to be audited 'a person or organisation must transform itself into an auditable commodity' (Shore and Wright, 1999: 570, quoted in Ball, 2006: 152). However, the voices of these young people revealed that fabrications conceal as much as they reveal. They are, as Ball (*ibid.*: 53) says, 'ways of presenting ourselves within particular registers of meaning, within a particular economy of meaning, in which only certain possibilities of meaning have value'. The young people in our study did not have the choice or the authority, nor necessarily the desire, to opt out altogether from the potential rewards of meeting performative ideals. Their fabrications were, therefore, 'deeply para-doxical', constituting, on the one hand, 'a way of eluding or deflecting direct surveillance as they provided a façade of calculation between the individual and her environment' through dieting in order to meet slender ideals. On the other hand, the work of fabricating the self required submission to the 'rigours and terms of performativity and the disciplines of competition'. This, then, was the unenviable position in which these middle-class young women found themselves as they literally embodied complicity while simultaneously rejecting the academic and health achievement criteria of performative ideals. The fabrications of the self they perpetrated offered both 'resistance and capitulation', constituting, in one sense, 'a betrayal even, a giving up of claims to authenticity and commitment, an investment in plasticity', in another, their only means of finding meaning and achieving some semblance of control over their lives. To the extent that per-formative meanings and criteria become embedded in and reproduced by systems of recording, reporting and practice – for example, in new regimes of weight measurement being implemented in UK schools – 'they also work to exclude other things (and people) which do not "fit" into what is intended to be represented or conveyed'. However, there is, as Ball points out, a paradox involving 'calculations which appear to make people more transparent [and] may actually result in making them more opaque as representational artefacts are increasingly constructed with great deliberation and sophistication'. Ironically, the more expert these young people became at meeting the performative ideals of popular culture, school and their peers, the less was seen of their 'authentic' selves. In search of meaning and significance, they took their corporeal actions to the extreme: 'now I am nobody, see me for who I really am'. As 'performance improvements' (in health and education) become the primary basis for their decision-making, it isn't just 'the heart of the educational project that is gouged out and left empty' but the deep ontological significance and meaning of those pupils and teachers who are compelled to pursue it. Thus, with fabrication of the self comes corrosion of the soul. 'Authenticity is replaced entirely by plasticity and the person becomes a suitable commodity'; these young people feel they are no more than transient indices of schools' performative ideals. It was hardly surprising that in the context of other life worries some became depressed and dangerously ill (all quotes from Ball, *ibid.*).

In many respects these young women are the embodiment of the postmodern condition, their identities reflections of 'external contingencies' (Bernstein, 2000a: 1942), dominant cultures and public issues. They lived within a culture in which there was a high degree of uncertainty and, like their teachers, they were, in Ball's (2006) terms, subject to myriad judgements, measures, comparisons and targets in contexts in which there was a high degree of uncertainty and instability, constantly calibrated in different ways by different means according to different criteria through different agents and agencies. For those who have little choice but to pursue schools' performative ideals and produce measurable and improving 'results' and performances, the inevitable consequences may be guilt, self-doubt, blame and shame. Even so, we repeat yet again, schools do not 'cause' eating disorders and nowhere do we, or the young people themselves, claim this to be so. But all refer repeatedly to (not 'causal' but 'contributory') relationships between their 'progress' towards disordered eating, excessive exercise and some of the prevailing health initiatives and messages in schools. Just as we should listen to the perspectives of obese, and indeed all, children and young people, so we should not be dismissive of the voices of those who have chosen to become excessively and dangerously thin, even if we do not like what they have to say. Too often their experiences are written off as revealing nothing about the culture in which we live but everything about their youthful psychiatric condition. Their voices, however, point to dangerous aspects of performativity and particularly the way in which academic and health discourse in a totally pedagogised micro-society commingle and intersect with the material and corporeal conditions of individuals' lives to create conditions of ill health. Like others working in the field of eating disorders, such as Gordon (2000), we have illustrated that it is the combination of stringent requirements for thinness within highly competitive environments that significantly elevates the risk of developing eating disorders. This dynamic, given the heavy emphasis on achievement and performance in the contemporary culture of schools in the UK and elsewhere, may be of considerable import to policy-makers and pedagogues, not least those promoting health education. The resultant cocktail of high-performance and body-centred pathology codes that we find in PE and other 'health' settings may have deeply damaging consequences for students' identity, education and health, particularly for those emotionally vulnerable and at risk. As we have seen, young people are vulnerable to being caught in the uncertainties and ambiguities of a fast-moving, global age. Complex interconnections between these aspects of schooling and other relationships and social practices within peer groups, families, paid and unpaid work and leisure need further interrogation, without which we are unlikely to help young people achieve the levels of control, responsibility and autonomy that they need if they are to avoid feeling alienated by formal education and some drifting towards disordered eating and ill health.

We have not in this study been able to explore these processes inside mainstream schools; indeed, that is a phase of research on which we are about to embark. Notwithstanding this limitation, the narratives of these young women do seem to endorse Ball's (2006) claim that performativity does not just get in the way of real academic work or proper learning but, rather, that it is a vehicle for changing what academic work and learning are and, critically, what 'the good person', whether student or teacher, ought to be when pursuing them. It involves fundamental changes in relationships between learners, learning and knowledge, resulting in what Ball describes as a thorough exteriorisation of the latter. Health knowledge and knowledge relations, including those between learners and their own bodies, can become de-socialised and deeply alienating. In such contexts young people may come to feel vulnerable, empty and either ignored or misrecognised for who they know they really are.

Endnote: where next?

Reading anorexia and other forms of serious body disaffection as discursive and material practices that are both self-productive and self-destructive tells us something significant about viable options for gaining control over one's identity in schools. These young women highlight a performative culture endorsed in school which builds pressure for perfection and performance, often in forms which are undesirable or impossible to achieve. Far from empowering individuals, social practices such as those described leave young people feeling powerless, alienated from their developing bodies and reaching towards starvation diets and obsessive exercise as means of regaining control over the base elements of their lives. The social injustice of placing such moral obligation and blame on individuals for their health problems in ways which depoliticise the roles that school and other social influences play in people's lives should be a major concern. We need clearer understanding of how various medical, social and spiritual understandings of 'normal' and emaciated bodies are appropriated, fused and legitimated within schooling. How is 'normality' delineated by wider social notions of what it means to be an individual or a 'middle-' or 'working-' class 'woman' or 'man', and how are they linked with career, family, relationships and other discourses? Insights on both would give a much stronger indication of the role schools play in the aetiology of eating disorders and other forms of corporeal disaffection, conditions which are as complex to account for as they are difficult to mend. In a fast-changing, post-modern world schools will have to address new expectations, new opportunities and gender relations and more attention will need to be paid to the micro-politics of power which are as significant as macro-formations. What is clear from the stories of these young people is that the complexity of social interaction in schools belies any simple notion of gender socialisation or reform strategy, such as critical-literacy or health-promotion strategies geared towards the treatment of single factors, such as weight or exercise, bearing on their lives. If nothing else, the data presented here should warrant a fundamental critique of any discourse that reduces the contribution of education to a trivium of food (diet), exercise and weight management or generates social practices in which children or young persons are reduced to 'bodies', not persons whose circumstances need to be understood if their health and educational requirements are to be met. To accept that there is no alternative to contemporary discourse of health or that there is and can be nothing new is, as Fitzpatrick (2001: 160–1) has observed, a recipe not only for ineffective health measures but for the stagnation of society and diminished expectations for the future:

> If collective aspirations are no longer viable, then the scope for individual aspirations is also reduced. The contemporary preoccupation with the body is one consequence of this [. . .] Once you give up on any prospect of achieving progress in society, your horizons are reduced to securing your own physical survival [. . .] From this perspective, quantitative indicators of health (of the individual and of society) become more important than indicators of the

quality of life. 'Life expectancy' – measured in units of time – becomes more important than any concern about how the additional time gained might be spent [. . .] If people's lives are ruled by the measures they believe may help to prolong their existence, the quality of their lives is diminished. The tyranny of health means the ascendancy of the imperatives of biology over the aspirations of the human spirit.

This presents educationalists and health education with something of a conundrum. Critical pedagogues do need to engage with the changing world in which health discourse is configured; it is not enough to criticise, explain or understand it. We have to engage with the paradox of wanting to reject utterly the performative values that are driving social change while at least considering that there also might be an immediate problem to deal with in the form of poor diet, too few opportunities for play and exercise, and ill health, and their origins in the social conditions of people's lives in a context of global capitalism. Critical pedagogy does not occur in a vacuum; as Apple (2006) reminds us, unless we honestly confront neo-liberal-inspired market proposals and neo-liberal purposes and think tactically about them we will have little effect either on the creation of counter-hegemonic common sense, in this case about health, or on the building of counter-hegemonic alliances. Certainly our analyses have, as Apple implores, to be sufficiently connected to the ways in which conservative modernisation has altered common sense, including that relating to health and transformed the material and ideological conditions surrounding schooling. It also has to be aware of alternative belief systems and conceptions of 'health' and strategies for effecting the latter that might be drawn on while contesting the current orthodoxies of health policy and school pedagogic modalities. In view of this, to suggest that we reduce our analysis of 'health' to weight and exercise issues is at best limited and at worst patently absurd.

Appendix

The young women in the study (all of whom have been given pseudonyms) were aged between eleven and twenty, were white, of UK origin, able-bodied, and all had been diagnosed as 'having an eating disorder' (either anorexia nervosa or bulimia nervosa). Reflecting a wider demography of eating disorders (see Doyle and Bryant-Waugh, 2000), the majority of those attending the centre came from 'middle-class' families and had attended what might be described as 'high-status' comprehensive, grammar or private schools in various parts of the UK. The centre also accepted young men but received very few. At the time of study none were available for inclusion in the research. Operating rather like a boarding school, the centre provided compulsory, full-time education for residents while liaising with their schools to ensure continuity of work and to reduce anxieties concerning re-entry to mainstream education. Ethical clearance gained from the university supporting the research recognised that we were dealing with 'vulnerable young people' and that procedures required not only the full support and cooperation of centre staff but use of research techniques that were, above all else, sensitive to participants' health interests. Only after permission was granted from all parties concerned – the young people, parents and centre staff, including its resident psychiatrist and director – did data collection commence. All fieldwork (some involving periods of residential stay at the centre) was conducted by a female member of the research team (Rachel Allwood, abbreviated to RA in some of the transcripts that appear here) in the interest of building trust and rapport with participants. A variety of techniques – for example, formal and informal interviews, diary keeping, focus groups, field notes, email correspondence and mapping – was used to register participants' stories of how formal mainstream education figured in the development of their disordered behaviours and relationships with their own and others' bodies. Interviews were mostly of an informal nature, with much data being generated through conversations with the young people in their leisure time between other timetabled activities (e.g., education and counselling) which made up their day. The majority of participants were forthcoming with their views, relishing opportunities to speak of their previous school experience either directly or later using email communication. Participants also kept diaries to which they gave us access. Furthermore, we interviewed teachers who worked at the centre (who were also given pseudonyms). Data analyses followed the conventions of interpretative 'ethnographic' research. Categories and themes were allowed to emerge from the data, inform our sociological interests and guide our developing conceptual schema. It was agreed that the name and location of the clinic could be revealed.

Notes

1 Introduction

1 An eating disorder is defined as a 'persistent disturbance of eating or eating-related behaviour that results in the altered consumption of food and that significantly impairs physical health and/or psychological functioning' (Fairburn and Walsh, 1995: 135). Anorexia nervosa and bulimia nervosa are clinically defined by diagnostic criteria, most commonly those established by the American Psychiatric Association's *Diagnostic and Statistical Manual* (*DSM-IV-TR*; 2000). The former involves: refusal to maintain body weight over a minimum, normal weight for age and height; intense fear of gaining weight or becoming fat, even though underweight; disturbance in the way in which body weight, size or shape is experienced; restriction of food intake; and the presence of amenorrhoea. Bulimia nervosa involves recurrent episodes of binge eating, or recurrent, inappropriate compensatory behaviour to prevent weight gain, such as self-induced vomiting, misuse of laxatives, diuretics or other medications, fasting, or excessive exercise. A large volume of literature suggests that both conditions involve association of negative body image, fear of fat and feeling powerless and insecure (Levine and Piran, 1999: 321) and have strong risk periods during adolescence. These clinically defined eating disorders are, therefore, categorised as serious psychiatric illnesses, anorexia nervosa presenting itself as having one of the highest rates of mortality for any psychiatric condition, estimated at around 13–20 per cent per annum (Howlett *et al.*, 1995) in the UK. The *DSM-IV-TR* also highlights the condition of 'eating disorder not otherwise specified (EDNOS) characterised by those disturbed behaviors that do not meet all of the criteria needed to qualify as either anorexia or bulimia' (American Psychiatric Association, 2000: 594).

2 We emphasise that although our analysis is built on the accounts of young people who have taken extreme action with regard to weight, behaviour that few others would consider or endorse, their perspectives foreground the cultural toxins in schools and wider society that all pupils endure and which may underlie rising levels of alienation and body disaffection now apparent among very many young people. In short, we claim they speak for all children, as well as representing the voice of the vulnerable few. While relatively few people are impelled to take the dramatic actions of the girls in this study towards self-starvation, they reveal features of weight representation in schools to which many young people are subjected and which may underlie increasing levels of 'body disaffection' and 'dissatisfaction' now reported in Western societies (Grogan, 1999). Indeed, over the last few years, increasing 'medical' recognition has been given to a range of weight-related conditions which, while not defined as clinical 'eating disorders', point towards the prevalence of disordered eating of various kinds. Young people with such conditions are seen to exhibit disordered forms of eating or weight loss which might not meet the strict diagnostic criteria defined by *DSM-IV-TR*. Such disordered eating behaviours, rather than clinically defined eating disorders,

include *orthorexia*, an obsession with eating healthy foods, and *anorexia athletica* which involves compulsive over-exercising, often alongside restrictions on food intake. Our message, therefore, is that it is not just those who might be considered in psychiatric terms to be damaged or troubled in some ways who are prone to the dangers of obesity discourse. There are vast numbers of young people who do not experience clinically defined eating disorders yet continue to experience disordered relationships with food and the body as described above.

3   'A code is a regulative principle, tacitly acquired, which selects and integrates . . . meanings, realisations, contexts', later refined as 'orientations to meanings; textual productions, and specialised interactional practices' (Bernstein, 1990: 14). Perfection codes determine what bodily acts are permitted and forbidden, the positive and negative values of different possible behaviours of and on the body. They determine and define simultaneously 'what "the body" is and ideally ought to be' (Evans and Davies, 2004: 215).

2 Body pedagogies, obesity discourse and disordered eating

1

The BMI ranges	
Underweight	Under 18.5
Normal range	between 18.5–24.9
Overweight	between 25–29.9
Obese class 1	30–34.9
Obese class 2	35–39.9
Obese class 3	40 and over

Source: Adapted from WHO (2004)

Note: Body Mass Index is calculated by dividing weight in kilograms by height in metres squared.

3 Sacred knowledge, science and health policy

1   When quoting interviewees, we use '. . .' to indicate a significant pause in the interview and '[. . .]' when we have edited what was said.

2   It is worth reminding ourselves here of Steven Blair's broadside on the Institute of Medicine report's new dietary recommendations, in which he claims:

> The amount of physical activity required for maximal or optimal health benefits is unclear. We also are uncertain about the amount of activity necessary to prevent weight gain, and there is extensive individual variation. For example, some individuals never exercise yet also do not gain any weight during their adult years, while others gain a substantial amount of weight despite daily jogging, such as a certain ageing epidemiologist at The Cooper Institute.
> (Blair comments reported on 23 September 2002 via the Australian Physical
> Education Discussion List: http.//www.austpe-1@hms.uq.edu.au)

3   More sanguine and cautious voices are barely heard (Gaessor, 2003). Brodney *et al.* (2000), for example, have suggested that programmes concentrating on weight and dietary change are not only seriously limited in their foci but are not working. Their painstaking research on the overweight and obese suggests that 'men who were unfit

had a higher relative risk for all-cause mortality than their fit peers at all body fatness and waist circumference categories' (*ibid.*: 365). In short, size is not the issue: 'Obese men who are at least moderately fit (physically active) do not have an elevated mortality rate and, in fact, this group had a much lower death rate than unfit men in the <27 BMI category (18.0 compared with 52.1 deaths per 10,000)' (*ibid.*). They argue that 'public health would be better served with more comprehensive attempts to increase population levels of physical activity, rather than emphasising ideal weight and ranges and raising an alarm about increasing prevalence rates of obesity' (*ibid.*: 367). Thus, although overweight and obesity are constructed as pathological, for many patients there might be little or no relation between their weight and health. The relationships between obesity and health are more tenuous, complex and contradictory than the obesity-epidemic discourse would lead us to believe (Gard and Wright, 2001).

5 Popular pedagogies

1 There is not space to detail further the various studies which contest the reliability of BMI for assessing one's health. However, Campos cites what he describes as 'one of the most comprehensive surveys of the literature regarding the health risks of different weight levels' – a study by scientists at the National Center for Health Statistics and Cornell University (Troiano *et al.*, 1996). This survey analysed data from dozens of previous studies involving more than 600,000 subjects. It concluded that, for non-smoking men, the lowest mortality rate was found among those with BMI figures between 23 and 29, meaning that a large majority of the healthiest men in the survey would be considered 'overweight' by BMI standards. For non-smoking women, it was concluded that the BMI range correlating with the lowest mortality rate is extremely broad, from about 18 to 32. Any woman lying in this range would not see 'any statistically meaningful change in her risk of premature death' (Campos, 2004: 12).

6 Solving the obesity crisis?

1 The same cannot be said of PE and sport in primary schools in the UK. In this sector, the relative absence of specialist PE teachers and limited training in either PE or sport given to generalist classroom teachers combine with pressures to meet literacy and numeracy targets to ensure that both their quality and quantity in schools' timetables is sometimes very limited (see Caldecott *et al.*, 2006).

2 In any field, the manner in which legitimate knowledge is assembled and transmitted is a systematic activity whose rules are expressions of society's wider distribution of power and control. While knowledge may exist *sui generis* as disciplines, school subjects are their delocated versions whose form and content changes. Bernstein (1996, 2001) noted that while their singular forms (maths, English, science, modern languages, history, etc.) are remarkably resilient, particularly in our secondary schools, new ones arise and new combinations are brought into existence as curricular regions and generic forms – represented, for example, in schools and further education by National Council for Vocational Qualifications (NCVQ) pedagogic and assessment modes – which privilege policy commitment to the primacy of the 'needs of industry' for flexible, competence-based 'trainability'. While clearly generic vocationally oriented curricular forms have long been staples of further and higher education, from medicine to carpentry, we have required primary and secondary teachers to learn on their feet as policy-makers decree new curricular content and assessment formats, and successively prescribing models of pedagogic practice that are either competence- or performance-based (see Fitz *et al.*,2006, particularly chs. 1 and 6).

3 Since the 1980s in the UK (and elsewhere, see Bonal and Rambla, 2003) the state has effectively colonised the pedagogical recontextualising field (PRF) by a process of appropriation of specific pedagogic discourses and the production of new curriculum

policy (in the UK, for example, the NCPE). The relative autonomy of the PRF has been weakened by extension and growth of the official recontextualising field (ORF) through 'co-option practices' (*ibid*.: 176; see also Chapter 7, this volume). Leading figures ('experts') from the worlds of sport and health have been successfully incorporated into the state apparatus to advise on, among other things, both the form and content of PE and health education in schools. Although these processes have not happened without struggle and are not without contradiction (see Penney and Evans, 1999), they have effectively meant the privileging of particular pedagogical orientations: performance (generic) and perfection codes and their manifestation in the dominance of sport/games teaching and fitness and health education in the PE curriculum.

7 Class, control and embodiment

1 Butler and Savage (1995: vii) point out that 'traditionally the social scientific gaze has been directed either downwards, to the working classes, the poor and the dispossessed, or upwards, to the wealthy and powerful'. Power (2000), on the other hand, suggests that a possible reason for the relative neglect of the middle class might be its problematic location within conventional class theory and, in particular, the extent to which it is subsumed within other debates (see also Skeggs, 1997). And only recently has a body of feminist work begun to (re-)emerge, which counts class as a 'difference which makes a difference' (Coole, 1996; Lawler, 1999).

10 Health education, weight management or social control?

1 In Australia, health promotion has most recently been pursued through such government publications as *Healthy Weight 2008: Australia's Future* (Commonwealth of Australia, 2003). A British equivalent would be *Every Child Matters* (DfES, 2003).

Bibliography

Alderson, P. (1995) *Listening to Children: Children, Ethics and Social Research*, Ilford: Barnados.

Aldrich, R., Kemp, L., Harris, E., Simpson, S., Wilson, A., McGill, K., Byles, J., Lowe, J. and Jackson, T. (2003) Using Socioeconomic Evidence in Clinical Practice Guidelines, *British Medical Journal*, 327: 1283–1285.

American Psychiatric Association (2000) *Diagnostic and Statistical Manual of Mental Disorders*, 4th revised edn (*DSM-IV-TR*), Washington, DC: American Psychiatric Association.

Antonovosky, A. (1979) *Health, Stress and Coping*, San Francisco, CA: Jossey-Bass.

—— (1996) The Salutogenic Model as a Theory to Guide Health Promotion, *Health Promotion International*, 11 (1): 11–18.

Aphramor, L. (2005) Is a Weight-centred Health Framework Salutogenic? Some Thoughts on Unhinging Certain Dietary Ideologies, *Social Theory and Health*, 3 (4): 315–340.

—— (2006) Scales before Our Eyes: Fatness as if Social Justice Mattered, paper presented at Expanding the Obesity Debate Conference, Limerick, Ireland, 9 January.

Apple, M. (2006) Producing Inequalities: Neo-liberalism, Neo-conservativism, and the Politics of Educational Reform, in H. Lauder., P. Brown., J-A. Dillabough and A.H. Halsey (eds) *Education, Globalisation and Social Change*, Oxford: Oxford University Press.

Armstrong, N. (1990) *New Directions in Physical Education*, Vol. 1, Leeds: Human Kinetics.

—— (1992) *New Directions in Physical Education*, Vol. 2, Leeds: Human Kinetics.

Armstrong, N. and Sparkes, S. (1991) *Issues in Physical Education*, Trowbridge: Cassell.

Arnot, M. and Reay, D. (2006) Power, Pedagogic Voices and Pupil Talk: The Implications for Pupil Consultation as Transformative Practice, in R. Moore, M. Arnot, J. Beck and H. Daniels (eds) *Knowledge, Power and Educational Reform*, London: Routledge**.**

Atrens, D. (2000) *The Power of Pleasure*, Sydney: Duffy and Snellgrove.

Austin, S.B. (1999) Fat, Loathing and Public Health: The Complicity of Science in a Culture of Disordered Eating, *Culture, Medicine and Psychiatry*, 23: 245–268.

Azzarito, L. (2008) The Rise of Corporate Curriculum: Fatness, Fitness, and Whiteness, in J. Wright and V. Harwood (eds) *Bio-Pedagogies: Schooling, Youth and the Body in the 'Obesity Epidemic'*, London: Routledge.

Azzarito, L. and Solmon, M.A. (2006) A Poststructural Analysis of High School Students' Gender and Racialized Bodily Meanings, *Journal of Teaching in Physical Education*, 25, 75–98.

Ball, S.J. (1990) *Politics and Policy Making in Education*, London: Routledge.

—— (2003a) *Class Strategies and the Education Market: The Middle Classes and Social Advantage*, London: RoutledgeFalmer.

—— (2003b) The Teacher's Soul and the Terrors of Performativity, *Journal of Education Policy*, 18 (2): 215–228.

—— (2004a) Performativities and Fabrications in the Education Economy: Toward the Performative Society, in S.J. Ball (ed.) *The RoutledgeFalmer Reader in Sociology of Education*, London: RoutledgeFalmer.

—— (2004b) *Professionalism, Managerialism and Performativity*, London: Institute of Education, University of London.

—— (2006) *Education Policy and Social Class*, London: Routledge.

—— (2007a) *Education plc: Understanding Private Sector Participation in Public Sector Education*, London: Routledge

—— (2007b) 'Going Further': Tony Blair and New Labour Education Policies, working paper, London: Institute of Education.

Ball, S.J., Bowe, R. and Gewirtz, S. (1996) School Choice, Social Class and Distinction: The Realization of Social Advantage in Education, *Journal of Education Policy*, 11: 89–112.

BBC News Online (2000) Eating Disorders. Available at: http://news.bbc.co.uk/1/hi/health/medical_notes/1079435.stm (accessed 20 December 2000).

—— (2006) Baby Growth Charts to be Revised. Available at: http://news.bbc.co.uk/1/hi/health/4938234.stm (accessed 24 April 2006).

Beat (2007) Understanding Eating Disorders. Available at: http//www.beat.co.uk/ProfessionalStudentResources/Studentinformation-1/SomeStatistics (accessed 26 October 2007).

Beck, U. and Beck-Gernsheim, E. (2006) Beyond Status and Class, in H. Lauder, P. Brown, J-A Dillabough and A.H. Halsey (eds) *Education, Globalisation and Social Change*, Oxford: Oxford University Press.

Becker, H.S. (1971) Becoming a Marihuana User, in B. Cosin, I. Dale, G. Esland and D.F. Swift (eds) *School and Society*, London: Routledge and Kegan Paul in association with the Open University Press.

Beckett, L. (2004) Special Issue: Health, the Body, and Identity Work in Health and Physical Education, *Sport, Education and Society*, 9 (2): 171–175.

Beckett-Milburn, K. (2000) Parents, Children and the Construction of the Healthy Body in Middle Class Families, in A. Prout (ed.) *The Body, Childhood and Society*, London: Palgrave Macmillan.

Bernstein, B. (1971) On the Classification and Framing of Educational Knowledge, in M.F.D. Young (ed.) *Knowledge and Control: New Directions for the Sociology of Education*, London: Collier Macmillan.

—— (1990) *The Structuring of Pedagogic Discourse*, Vol. 4: *Class, Codes and Control*, London: Routledge.

—— (1996) *Pedagogy, Symbolic Control and Identity*, London: Taylor & Francis.

—— (2000a) Offical Knowledge and Pedagogic Identities: The Politics of Recontextualisation, in S.J. Ball (ed.) The *Sociology of Education: Major Themes*, London: Routledge.

—— (2000b) *Pedagogy, Symbolic Control and Identity*, Boston: Rowman & Littlefield.

—— (2001) From Pedagogies to Knowledges, in A. Morias, I. Neves, B. Davies and H. Daniels (eds) *Towards a Sociology of Pedagogy: The Contribution of Basil Bernstein to Research*, New York: Peter Lang.

Blackman, L. (1996) The Dangerous Classes: Retelling the Psychiatric Story, *Feminism and Psychology*, 6 (3) (special issue on social class): 355–379.

Board of Education (BoE) (1933) *Syllabus of Physical Training for Schools*, London: Her Majesty's Stationery Office.

Boero, N. (2007) All the News that's Fat to Print: The American 'Obesity Epidemic' and the Media, *Qualitative Sociology*, 30: 41–46.

Boler, M. and Zembylas, M. (2003) Discomforting Truths: The Emotional Terrain of Understanding Differences, in P. Tryfonas (ed.) *Pedagogies of Difference: Rethinking Education for Social Justice*, New York: Routledge.

Bonal, X. and Rambla, X. (2003) Captured by the Totally Pedagogised Society: Teachers and Teaching in the Knowledge Economy, *Globalisation, Societies and Education*, 1 (2): 169–184.

Bordo, S. (1993) *Unbearable Weight: Feminism, Western Culture and the Body*, London: University of California Press.

Borsay, P. (2007) Binge Drinking and Moral Panics, paper presented at the Addressing Binge Drinking: Challenges and Opportunities Conference, London School of Hygiene and Tropical Medicine, 14 February.

Bouchard, C. (2000) Introduction, in C. Bouchard (ed.) *Physical Activity and Health*, Champaign, IL: Human Kinetics.

Bouchard, C. and Blair, S.N. (1999) Introductory Comments for the Consensus on Physical Activity and Obesity, *Medicine and Science in Sports Science*, 31 (11) (Suppl.): S498–S501.

Bourdieu, P. (1978) Sport and Social Class, *Social Science Information*, 17: 819–840.

—— (1986) The Forms of Social Capital, in J. Richardson (ed.) *Handbook of Theory and Research for the Sociology of Education*, New York: Greenwood Press.

Bray, A. (1994) The Edible Woman: Reading/Eating Disorders and Femininity, *Media Information Australia*, 72: 4–10.

Brink, P.J. (1994) Stigma and Obesity, *Clinical Nursing Research*, 3 (4): 291–293.

British Heart Foundation (BHF) (1999) *Overweight, Obesity and Cardiovascular Disease*, London: British Heart Foundation.

British Medical Journal (2004) Select Committee Castigated for Citing Death of 3 Year Old Girl in Obesity Report, 19 June. Available at: http://www.bmj.com/cgi/content/full/328/7454/1503 (accessed 18 May 2007).

Brodney, S., Blair, S.N. and Lee, C.D. (2000) Is it Possible to be Overweight and Fit and Healthy?, in C. Bouchard (ed.) *Physical Activity and Health*, Champaign, IL: Human Kinetics.

Brown, P. (1988) *The Body and Society*, London: Faber and Faber.

Brown, P. and Hesketh, A. (2004) *The Management of Talent: Employability and Jobs in the Knowledge Economy*, Oxford: Oxford University Press.

Brownell, K.D. (1995) Definition and Classification of Obesity, in K.D. Brownell and C.G. Fairburn (eds) *Eating Disorders and Obesity: A Comprehensive Handbook*, New York: The Guilford Press.

Brownell, K.D., Puhl, R.M., Schwartz, M.B. and Rudd, L. (2005) *Weight Bias: Nature Consequences, and Remedies*, London: The Guilford Press.

Bruch, H. (1973) *Eating Disorders: Obesity, Anorexia and the Person Within*, Houston, TX: Basic Books.

Bryant-Waugh, R. (2000) Overview of the Eating Disorders, in B. Lask and R. Bryant-Waugh (eds) *Anorexia Nervosa and Related Eating Disorders in Childhood and Adolesence*, 2nd edn, London: Psychology Press.

Bunton, R. (1997) Popular Health, Advance Liberalism and Good Housekeeping, in A. Petersen and R. Bunton (eds) *Foucault, Health and Medicine*, New York: Routledge.

Bunton, R. and Burrows, R. (1995) Consumption and Health in the 'Epidemiological' Clinic of Late Modern Medicine, in R. Bunton, S. Nettleton and R. Burrows (eds) *The Sociology of Health Promotion*, London and New York: Routledge.

Burke, A. (1983) New Languages: Power, Feeling, Communication, *Borderlands E-Journal*, 2 (3). Available at: http://www.borderlandsejournal.adelaide.edu.au/vol2no3_2003/burke_editorial.htm (accessed 6 February 2008).

Burman , E. (2005) Childhood, Neo-liberalism and the Feminization of Education, *Gender and Education*, 17 (4): 351–367.

Burrows, L. and Wright, J. (2004a) The Discursive Production of Childhood, Identity and Health, in J. Evans, B. Davies and J. Wright (eds) *Body Knowledge and Control*, London: Routledge.

—— (2004b) The Good Life: New Zealand's Children's Perspectives on Health and Self, *Sport, Education and Society*, 9 (2): 193–207.

—— (2007) Prescribing Practices: Shaping Healthy Children in Schools, *International Journal of Children's Rights*, 15: 83–98.

Burry, J.N. (1999) Obesity and Virtue: Is Staying Lean a Matter of Ethics?, *Medical Journal Australia*, 171: 609–610.

Butler, J. (1990) *Gender Trouble, Subversion and the Foundation of Identity*, New York: Routledge.

—— (1993) *Bodies that Matter: On the Discursive Limits of Sex*, New York: Routledge.

—— (1994) Gender as Performance, *Radical Philosophy*, 67, 32–39.

—— (1997) *The Psychic Life of Power: Theories of Subjection*, Stanford, CA: Stanford University Press.

Butler, T. and Savage, M. (1995) *Social Change and the Middle Class*, London: UCL Press.

Bynum, C.W. (1987) *Holy Feast and Holy Fast: The Religious Significance of Food to Medieval Women*, Berkeley: University of California Press.

Caldecott, S., Warburton, P. and Waring, M. (2006) A Survey of the Time Devoted to the Preparation of Primary and Junior School Trainee Teachers to Teach Physical Education in England, *Physical Education Matters*, 1 (1): 45–48.

Campos, P. (2004) *The Obesity Myth*, New York: Gotham Books.

Campos, P., Saguy, A., Ernberger, P., Oliver, E. and Gaesser, G. (2006) The Epidemiology of Overweight and Obesity: Pubic Health Crisis or Moral Panic?, *International Journal of Epidemiology*, 35 (1): 55–60.

Cant, S. and Sharma, U. (2000) Alternative Health Practices and Systems, in G. Albrecht, R. Fitzpatrick and S. Scrimshaw (eds) *Handbook of Social Studies in Health and Medicine*, London: Sage.

Carlyle, D. and Woods, P. (2002) *Emotions of Teacher Stress*, London: Trentham.

Carryer, J. (1997) The Embodied Experience of Largeness, in M. de Ras and V. Grace (eds) *Bodily Boundaries, Sexualised Genders and Medical Discourses*, New Zealand: Dunmore Press.

—— (2001) Embodied Largeness: A Significant Women's Health Issue, *Nursing Inquiry*, 8: 90–97.

Chatman, S. (1978) *Story and Discourse*, Ithaca, NY: Cornell University Press.

Cheniss, C. and Goleman, D. (2001) *The Emotionally Intelligent Work Place*, San Francisco, CA: Jossey-Bass.

Chomsky, N. (2005) *Imperial Ambitions*, London: Penguin.

Christensen, P. and James, A. (2000) *Research with Children: Perspectives and Practices*, London: Falmer.

Clark, L. (2007) Jamie's Healthy Meals Turn off 400,000 Pupils, *Daily Mail*, 4 September.

Cogan, J. (1999) Re-evaluating the Weight Centred Approach toward Health: The Need for a Paradigm Shift, in J. Sobal and D. Maurer (eds) *Interpreting Weight: The Social Management of Fatness and Thinness*, New York: Aldine De Gruyter.

Commonwealth of Australia (2003) *Healthy Weight 2008: Australia's Future*, Canberra: Department of Health and Ageing.

Connolly, C. and Corbett, D.P. (1990) Eating Disorders: A Framework for School Nursing Initiatives, *Journal of School Health*, 60 (8): 401–415.

Coole, D. (1996) Is Class a Difference that Makes a Difference?, *Radical Philosophy*, 77: 17–25.

Crawford, R. (1980) Healthism and the Medicalisation of Everyday Life, *International Journal of Health Sciences*, 10 (3): 365–389.

Daigneault, S.D. (2000) Body Talk: A School Based Group Intervention for Working with Disordered Eating Behaviours, *Journal for Specialists in Group Work*, 25 (2): 191–213.

Daily Express (2004) Child 3 Dies from Being too Fat, 27 May.

Daily Mirror (2004a) A Big Fat Lie, 10 June.

—— (2004b) War on Obesity: Docs Fight New Black Death, 12 March.

Daily Telegraph (2006) Anti-obesity Squad at the Door. Available at: http://www.news. com.au/dailytelegraph/story/0,22049,20643254-5006007,00.html (accessed 26 October 2006).

Davidson, F. (2007) Childhood Obesity Prevention and Physical Activity in Schools, *Health Education*, 107 (4): 377–395.

Davies, B. (2004a) Identity, Abjection and Otherness: Creating the Self, Creating Difference, *International Journal for Equity and Innovation in Early Childhood*, 2 (1): 58–80.

—— (2004b) Introduction: Poststructuralist Lines of Flight in Australia, *International Journal of Qualitative Studies in Education*, 17 (1): 3–9.

Davis, Z. (2004) The Debt to Pleasure: The Subject and Knowledge in Pedagogic Discourse, in J. Muller, B. Davies and A. Morais (eds) *Reading Bernstein, Researching Bernstein*, London: RoutledgeFalmer.

Dawson, A. (1994) Professional Codes of Practices and Ethical Conduct, *Journal of Applied Philosophy*, 11: 145–153.

Dean, M. (1995) Governing the Unemployed Self in an Active Society, *Economy and Society*, 24: 559–583.

Deleuze, G. and Guattari, F. (1987) *A Thousand Plateaus: Capitalism and Schizophrenia*, Minneapolis: University of Minnesota Press.

Department for Education and Science (DfES) (2003) *Every Child Matters*, London: HMSO.

Department of Health (2005a) *National Healthy School Status*, London: DoH Publications Orderline.

—— (2005b) Pubic Health White Paper, London: DoH Publications Orderline.

—— (2007) *Supporting Healthy Lifestyles: The National Child Measurement Programme*, London: HMSO.

Dixey, R., Sahota, P., Atwal, S. and Turner, A. (2001) Ha Ha You're Fat, We're Strong: A Qualitative Study of Boys' and Girls' Perceptions of Fatness and Thinness, Social Pressures and Health Using Focus Groups, *Health Education*, 101 (5): 206–211.

Douglas, M. (1970) *Natural Symbols*, London: Routledge.

Doyle, J. and Bryant-Waugh, R.A. (2000) Epidemiology, in B. Lask and R. Bryant-Waugh (eds) *Anorexia Nervosa and Related Eating Disorders in Childhood and Adolescence*, Hove: Psychology Press and Taylor & Francis.

Duncan, P. (2004) Dispute, Dissent and the Place of Health Promotion in a 'Disrupted Tradition' of Health Improvement, *Public Understanding of Science*, 13: 177–190.

Durkheim, E. (1995 [1912]) *The Elementary Forms of Religious Life*, New York: Free Press.

Eckerman, T. (1997) Foucault, Self-starvation and Gendered Subjectivities, in A. Petersen and R. Bunton (eds) *Foucault, Health and Medicine*, London: Routledge.

Edgley, C. and Brissett, D. (1999) *A Nation of Meddlers*, Boulder, CO: Westview Press.

Egger, G. and Swinburn, B. (1997) An 'Ecological' Approach to the Obesity Pandemic, *British Medical Journal*, 315: 477–480.

Emmons, L. (1994) Predisposing Factors Differentiating Adolescent Dieters and Non-dieters, *Journal of American Dieticians Association*, 94: 725–731.

Evans, B. (2007) Doing More Good than Harm – Every Child Matters? The Absent Presence of Children's Bodies in (Anti)Obesity Policy, paper presented at Society for Education Studies Conference, Loughborough University, September.

Evans, J. (2003) Physical Education and Health: A Polemic, or, Let Them Eat Cake!, *European Physical Education Review*, 9: 87–103.

Evans, J. and Davies, B. (2004) The Embodiment of Consciousness: Bernstein, Health and Schooling, in J. Evans, B. Davies and J. Wright (eds) *Body Knowledge and Control*, London: Routledge.

Evans, J., Davies, B. and Wright, J. (2004a) *Body Knowledge and Control: Studies in the Sociology of Physical Education and Health*, London: Routledge.

Evans, J., Rich, E. and Davies, B. (2004b) The Emperor's New Clothes: Fat, Thin and Overweight: The Social Construction of Risk and Ill-health, *Journal of Teaching in Physical Education*, 23: 372–391.

Evans, J., Rich, E. and Holroyd, R. (2004c) Disordered Eating and Disordered Schooling: What Schools Do to Middle Class Girls, *British Journal of Sociology of Education*, 25: 123–143.

Evans, J., Evans, R., Evans, C. and Evans, J.E. (2002a) Fat Free Schooling: The Discursive Production of Ill-health, *International Studies in the Sociology of Education*, 12 (2): 191–212.

Evans, J., Evans, B. and Rich, E. (2002b) Eating Disorders and Comprehensive Ideals, *Forum for Promoting 3–19 Comprehensive Education*, 44: 59–66.

Evans, J., Rich, E., Allwood, R. and Davies, B. (2008) Body Pedagogies, P/policy, Health and Gender, *British Educational Research Journal*, 34 (4): in press.

Fairburn, C.G. and Walsh, B.T. (1995) Atypical Eating Disorders, in K.D. Brownell and C.G. Fairburn (eds) *Eating Disorders and Obesity: A Comprehensive Handbook*, New York: The Guilford Press.

Fallon, P.A., Katzman, M. and Wooley, S.C. (1994) *Feminist Perspectives of Eating Disorders*, New York: The Guilford Press.

Featherstone, M. (1991) The Body in Consumer Culture, in M. Featherstone, M. Hepworth and B. Turner (eds) *The Body: Social Processes and Cultural Theory*, London: Sage.

Fikkan, J. and Rothblum, E. (2005) Weight Bias in Employment, in K.D. Brownell, R.M. Puhl, M.B. Schwartz and L. Rudd (eds) *Weight Bias: Nature, Consequences and Remedies*, New York: The Guilford Press.

Fitz, J., Davies, B. and Evans J. (2006) *Educational Policy and Social Reproduction*, London: Routledge.

Fitzpatrick, M. (2001) *The Tyranny of Health: Doctors and the Regulation of Lifestyle*, London: Routledge.

Flegal, K.M. (1999) The Obesity Epidemic in Children and Adults: Current Evidence and Research Issues, *Medicine and Science in Sports and Exercise*, 31: S509–S514.

Flegal, K.M., Graubard, B.L.,Williamson, D.F. and Gail, M.H. (2005) Excess Deaths Associated with Underweight, Overweight, and Obesity, *Journal of the American Medical Association*, 293: 1861–1867.

Foresight (2005) Tackling Obesities: Future Choice Projects. Available at: http://www.foresight.gov.uk/Obesity/Obesity.htm (accessed 27 March 2007).

—— (2007) *Tackling Obesities: Future Choices – Project Report*, London: Government Office for Science.

Foucault, M. (1972) *The Archaeology of Knowledge and the Discourse on Language*, London: Pantheon.

—— (1973) *The Birth of the Clinic*, London: Tavistock.

—— (1978) *The History of Sexuality*, Vol. 1: *An Introduction*, Harmondsworth: Peregrine, Penguin.

—— (1979) *Discipline and Punish*, London: Peregrine.

—— (1980) *Power/Knowledge: Selected Interviews and Other Writings 1972–1977*, ed. Colin Gordon, New York: Pantheon.

—— (1994) *The Birth of the Clinic: An Archaeology of Medical Perception*, New York: Vintage.

—— (2000) Governmentality, in J.D. Faubion (ed.) *Power, the Essential Works of Michel Foucault*, Vol. 3, New York: The New Press.

Fowles, J. (1996) *Advertising and Popular Culture*, London: Sage.

Fox, K.R. (1991) Physical Education and its Contribution to Health and Well-being, in N. Armstrong and A. Sparkes (eds) *Issues in Physical Education*, London: Cassell.

Frank, A. (1991) From Sick Role to Health Role: Deconstructing Parsons, in R. Robertson and B. Turner (eds) *Talcott Parsons*, London: Sage.

Frank, A.W (2006) Health Stories as Connectors and Subjectifiers, *Health: An Interdisciplinary Journal for the Social Study of Health, Illness and Medicine*, 10: 421–440.

Frost, L. (2001) *Young Women and the Body: A Feminist Sociology*, Basingstoke: Palgrave.

Furedi, F. (2007) Our Unhealthy Obsession with Sickness. Available at: http://www.spiked-online.com/Articles/0000000CA958.htm (accessed 19 March 2007).

Gabe, J. (1995) Health, Medicine and Risk, in J. Gabe (ed.) *Medicine, Health and Risk*, Oxford: Blackwell.

Gaessor, G.A. (2003) Is it Necessary to be Thin to be Healthy?, *Harvard Health Policy Review*, 4: 40–42.

Gard, M. (2004a) An Elephant in the Room and a Bridge too Far, or Physical Education and the 'Obesity Epidemic', in J. Evans, B. Davies and J. Wright (eds) *Body Knowledge and Control*, London: Routledge.

—— (2004b) Desperately Seeking Certainty: Statistics, Physical Activity and Critical Enquiry, in J. Wright, D. Macdonald and L. Burrows (eds) *Critical Inquiry and Problem Solving in Physical Education*, London: Routledge.

Gard, M. and Wright, J. (2001) Managing Uncertainty: Obesity Discourse and Physical Education in a Risk Society, *Studies in Philosophy and Education*, 20: 535–549.

—— (2005) *The Obesity Epidemic: Science, Morality and Ideology*, London: Routledge.

Gardner, H. (1993) *Multiple Intelligences: The Theory in Practice*, New York: Basic Books.

Garfinkel, E. and Garner, D.M. (1982) *Anorexia Nervosa: A Multidimensional Approach*, New York: Brunner Mazel.

Garland-Thomson, R. (2005) Feminist Disability Studies, *Signs, Journal of Women in Culture and Society*, 30 (2): 1557–1587.

Gastaldo, D. (1997). Is Health Education Good for You? Rethinking Health Education through the Concept of Bio-Power, in A. Petersen and R. Bunton (eds) *Foucault, Health and Medicine*, London: Routledge.

Geertz, C. (1983) *Local Knowledge: Further Essays in Interpretive Anthropology*, New York: Basic Books.

Gergen, M. and Gergen, K.J. (2003) Positive Ageing, in J. Gubrium and J.A. Holstein (eds) *Ways of Aging*, Oxford: Blackwell.

Giddens, A. (1973) *The Class Structure of Advanced Societies*, London: UCL Press.

—— (1991) *Modernity and Self-identity*, Cambridge: Polity Press.

—— (1998) Risk Society: The Context of British Politics, in J. Franklin (ed.) *The Politics of Risk Society*, Cambridge: Polity Press.

—— (1999) Reith Lectures. Available at: http://www.lse.ac.uk/Giddens/reith_99/week3/week3.htm (accessed 6 February 2008).

Giles, D.C. (2003) Narratives of Obesity as Presented in the Context of a Television Talk Show, *Journal of Health Psychology*, 8 (3): 317–326.

Gill, A.A. (2007) Jamie's Digging a Garden of Eden, *Sunday Times Culture*, 12 August.

Glaser, B. and Strauss, A. (1967) The *Discovery of Grounded Theory*, London: Weidenfeld and Nicolson.

Goffman, E. (1963) *Stigma: Notes on the Management of Spoiled Identity*, New York: Prentice-Hall.

Goldman, E.L. (1996) Eating Disorders on the Rise in Pre-teens, Adolescents, *Psychiatry News*, 24 (2): 10.

Goleman, D. (2000) *Working with Emotional Intelligence*, New York: Bantam.

Gordon, R.A. (2000) *Eating Disorders: Anatomy of an Epidemic*, Oxford: Blackwell.

—— (2001) Eating Disorders East and West: A Culture-bound Syndrome Unbound, in A. Nasser, M.N. Katzman and R.A. Gordon (eds) *Eating Disorders and Culture in Transition*, East Sussex: Brunner and Routledge.

Green, J. (1995) Accidents and the Risk Society, in R. Bunton, S. Nettleton and R. Burrows (eds) *The Sociology of Health Promotion*, London: Routledge.

Gregg, E.W., Cheng, Y.J., Cadwell, B.L., Imperatore, G., Williams, D.E., Flegal, K.M., Narayan, K.M. and Williamson, D.F. (2005) Secular Trends in Cardiovascular Disease Risk Factors According to Body Mass Index in US Adults, *Journal of the American Medical Association*, 293: 1868–1874.

Griggs, G. and Wheeler, K. (2006) Mind the Gap! The Implications for Undergraduates Studying Sport Science Related Degrees and Gaining Places on PGCE Courses, *British Journal of Teaching Physical Education*, 36 (4): 6–8.

Grogan, S. (1999) *Body Image: Understanding Body Dissatisfaction in Men, Women and Children*, London: Routledge.

Groskopf, B. (2005) The Failure of Bio-power: Interrogating the 'Obesity Crisis', *Journal for the Arts, Sciences and Technology*, 3 (1): 41–47.

Guardian (2002) Jonah Lomu is Fat, 17 September.

—— (2004) White Paper to Tackle Obesity, 3 February.

—— (2007) Study Reveals Stressed Out 7–11 Year Olds, 12 October.

Guardian Unlimited (2007) Obesity Crisis to Cost £45bn a Year. Available at: http://observer.guardian.co.uk/uk_news/stoty/0,,2190844,00.html (accessed 17 October 2007).

Hales, C. and Boughtwood, D. (2007) The Paradox of Virtue: (Re)thinking Deviance, Anorexia and Schooling, *Gender and Education*, 19 (2): 219–235.

Halse, C. (2007) The Bio-citizen: Virtual Discourses, BMI and Responsible Citizenship, paper presented at the Bio-pedagogies Conference, University of Wollongong, 25–27 January.

Hargreaves, A. (2003) *Teaching in a Knowledge Society*, Maidenhead: Open University Press.

Harjunen, H. (2003) Obesity as a Marginalized and Liminal Experience, paper presented at the Making Sense of Health, Illness and Disease Conference, St Hilda's College, Oxford, July.

Harwood, V. (2007) *Diagnosing 'Disorderly' Children : A Critique of Behaviour Disorder Discourses*, Abingdon: Routledge.

Heidegger, M. (with Eugen Fink) (1979) *Heraclitus Seminar*, Huntington: University of Alabama Press.

—— (1993 [1954]) The Question Concerning Technology', in D. Krell (ed.) *Martin Heidegger: Basic Writings,* London: Routledge.

Henriques, J., Holloway, W., Urwin, C., Venn, C. and Walkerdine, V. (1984) *Changing the Subject: Psychology, Social Regulation and Identity*, London: Methuen.

Hepworth, J. (1999) *The Social Construction of Anorexia Nervosa*, London: Sage.

Hewitt, M. (1983) Biopolitics and Social Policy: Foucault's Account of Welfare, *Theory, Culture and Society*, 2: 67–84.

Hewitt, P.L., Flett, G.L. and Ediger, E. (1995) Perfectionism Traits and Perfectionist Self-presentation in Eating Disorder Attitudes, Characteristics and Symptoms, *International Journal of Eating Disorders*, 18: 317–326.

Hodgetts, D. and Chamberlain, K. (1999) Medicalisation and the Depiction of Laypeople in Television Health Documentary, *Health*, 3: 317–333.

Holroyd, R. (2003) Fields of Experience: Young People's Constructions of Embodied Identities, Ph.D. thesis, Loughborough University.

Holstein, J. and Gubrium, J. (2000) *Constructing the Lifecourse*, 2nd edn, Lanham, MD: Rowman Altamira Press.

House of Commons (2001) Select Committee of Public Accounts Ninth Report: Tackling Obesity in England. Available at: http://www.publications.parliament.uk/pa/cm20001 02/cmselect/cmpubacc/421/42103.hm (accessed 6 February 2008).

Howlett, M., McClelland, L. and Crisp, A.H. (1995) The Cost of the Illness that Defies, *Postgraduate Medical Journal*, 71: 36–39.

Howson, A. (2004) *The Body in Society: An Introduction*, Oxford: Polity Press.

Ikeda, J. and Naworski, P. (1992) *Am I Fat? Helping Young Children Accept Differences in Body Size*, Santa Cruz, CA: ETR Associates.

Ikeda, J., Amy, N.K., Ernsberger, P., Gaesser, G.A., Berg, F.M., Clark, C.A., Parham, E.S. and Peters, P. (2005) The National Weight Control Registry: A Critique, *Journal of Nutrition Education Behaviour*, 37: 203–205.

Insight Media (2007) Physical Education on DVD and Video. Available at: www.Insight-Media.com (accessed 6 February 2008).

Ivinson, G. and Duveen, G. (2006) Children's Recontextualisations of Pedagogy, in R. Moore, M. Arnot, J. Beck and H. Daniels (eds) *Knowledge, Power and Educational Reform*, London: Routledge.

Jackson, P. (1995) The Case of Passive Smoking, in R. Bunton, S. Nettleton and R. Burrows (eds), *The Sociology of Health Promotion*, London: Routledge.

Jade, D. (2002) *Eating Disorders and the Media*, Surrey: National Centre for Eating Disorders. Available at: http://www.eating-disorders.org.uk/docs/media.doc (accessed 6 February 2008).

James, A. (1993) *Childhood Identities and Self and Social Relationships in the Experience of the Child*, Edinburgh: Edinburgh University Press.

—— (2000) Embodied Being(s): Understanding the Self and the Body in Childhood, in A. Prout (ed.) *The Body, Childhood and Society*, Basingstoke: Macmillan Press.

Jenkins, S. (2007) Public Services with a Heart, *TimesOnLine*. Available at: http://www.timesonline.co.uk/tol/comment/columnists/simon_jenkins/article1563712.ece (accessed 25 March 2007).

Johns, D.P. (2005) Recontextualising and Delivering the Biomedical Model as a Physical Education Curriculum, *Sport, Education and Society*, 11 (1): 69–84.

Jonas, S. (2002) A Healthy Approach to the 'Health at Any Size' Movement, *Healthy Weight Journal*, 16: 45–48.

Jones, B. (2007) Infants Being Treated for Obesity. Available at: http://news.bbc.co.uk/1/hi/health/6751991.stm (accessed 4 June 2007).

Kassirer, J.P. and Angell, M. (1998) Losing Weight: An Ill-fated New Year's Resolution, *New England Journal of Medicine*, 338: 52–54.

Katzman, M. (1997) Getting the Difference Right: It's Power not Gender that Matters, *European Eating Disorders Review*, 5: 71–74.

Katzman, M. and Lee, S. (1997) Beyond Body Image: The Integration of Feminist and Transcultural Theories in Understandings of Self-starvation, *International Journal of Eating Disorders*, 22: 385–394.

Kelly, P. (2007) Governing Individualized Risk Biographies: New Class Intellectuals and the Problem of Youth At-risk, *British Journal of Sociology of Education*, 28 (1): 39–53.

Kenway, J. and Bullen, E. (2001) *Consuming Children. Education – Entertainment – Advertising*, Maidenhead: Open University Press.

Kindlon, D. (2006) *Alpha Girls: Understanding the new American Girl and how She is Changing the World*, New York: Rodale Books.

Kirk, D. (1992) *Defining Physical Education*, London: The Falmer Press.

—— (1993) *The Body, Schooling and Culture*, Geelong: Deakin University Press.

—— (1999) Physical Culture, Physical Education and Relational Analysis, *Sport, Education and Society*, 4 (1): 63–75.

—— (2004) Towards a Critical History of the Body, Identity and Health: Corporeal Power and School Practices, in J. Evans, B. Davies and J. Wright (eds) *Body Knowledge and Control*, London: Routledge.

Kirkland, A. (2006) What's at Stake in Fatness as a Disability?, *Disability Studies Quarterly*, 26 (1). Available at: http://www.dsq-sds-archives.org/2006_winter_toc.html. (accessed 8 February 2008).

Klein, R. (1996) *Eat Fat*, New York: Pantheon Books.

Kleinman, A. (1992) Pain and Resistance: The Delegitimation and Relegitimation of Local Worlds, in M-J. Good, P. Brodwin, B. Good and A. Kleinman (eds) *Pain as Human Experience*, Berkeley: University of California Press.

Kumanyika, S., Jeffrey, R.W., Morabia, A., Rittenbaugh, C. and Antpatis, V.J. (2002) Report: Obesity Prevention: The Case for Action, *International Journal of Obesity*, 26: 425–436.

Lask, B. (2000) Aetiology, in B. Lask and R. Bryant-Waugh (eds) *Anorexia Nervosa and Related Eating Disorders in Childhood and Adolescence*, London: Taylor & Francis.

Lask, B. and Bryant-Waugh, R. (eds) (2000) *Anorexia Nervosa and Related Eating Disorders in Childhood and Adolescence*, London: Taylor & Francis.

Lauder, H., Brown, P., Dillabough, J.A. and Halsey, A.H. (eds) (2006) *Education, Globalisation and Social Change*, Oxford: Oxford University Press.

Lawler, S. (1999) Getting out and Getting away: Women's Narratives of Class Mobility, *Feminist Review*, autumn: 3–24.

Lawrence, R.G (2004) Framing Obesity: The Evolution of News Discourse on a Public Health Issue, *Harvard International Journal of Press/Politics*, 9 (3): 56–75.

Le Fanu, J. (1999) *The Rise and Fall of Modern Medicine*, London: Abacus.

Levine, M.P. and Piran, N. (1999) Reflections, Conclusion, Future Directions, in N. Piran, M.P. Levine and C. Steiner-Adair (eds) *Preventing Eating Disorders*, Philadelphia, PA: Brunner/Mazel.

Lucey, H. and Reay, D. (2002) Carrying the Beacon of Excellence: Social Class Differentiation and Anxiety at a Time of Transition, *Journal of Education Policy*, 17 (3): 321–336.

Lucey, H., Melody, J. and Walkerdine, V. (2003) Uneasy Hybrids: Psychosocial Aspects of Becoming Educationally Successful Working-class Young Women, *Gender and Education*, 15 (3): 285–299.

Lundy, K. and Gillard, J. (2003) *Tackling Obesity and Promoting Community Well Being: Labor's Plan for a Healthier and More Active Australia*, Victoria: Labor Party Policy Paper 014.

Lupton, D. (1994) *Medicine as Culture*, London: Sage.

—— (1995) *The Imperatives of Health: Public Health and the Regulated Body*, London: Sage.

—— (1996) *Food, the Body and the Self*, London: Sage.

—— (ed.) (1999) *Risk and Socio-cultural Theory: New Directions and Perspective*, Cambridge: Cambridge University Press.

Lynch, J. (2000) Income Inequality and Health: Expanding the Debate, *Social Sciences and Medicine*, 51: 1001–1005.

Lyons, A.C. and Willitt, S. (1999) From Suet Pudding to Superhero: Representaions of Men's Health for Women, *Health*, 3: 283–302.

Lyons, S. (2000) Examining Media Representations: Benefits for Health Psychology, *Journal of Health Psychology*, 5: 349–358.

MacIntyre, A. (1984) *After Virtue*, 2nd edn, Notre Dame, IN: University of Notre Dame Press.

MacSween, M. (1993) *Anorexic Bodies: A Feminist and Sociological Perspective on Anorexia Nervosa*, London: Routledge.

Malson, H. (1998) *The Thin Woman: Feminism, Poststructuralism and the Social Psychology of Anorexia Nervosa*, London: Routledge.

Masterman, L. (1990) *Teaching the Media*, New York: Routledge.

Maton, K. (2006) On Knowledge Structures and Knower Structures, in R. Moore, M. Arnot, J. Beck and H. Daniels (eds) *Knowledge, Power and Educational Reform*, London: Routledge.

Mauss, M. (1973 [1934]) Techniques of the Body, *Economy and Society*, 2: 70–88.

McCarthy, C. and Dimitriadis, G. (1999) Governmentality and the Sociology of Education: Media, Educational Policy and Politics of Resentment, in H. Lauder, P. Brown, J-A. Dillabough and A.H. Halsey (eds) *Education, Globalisation and Social Change*, Oxford: Oxford University Press.

McGinnis, J.M. and Foege, W.H. (1993) Actual Causes of Death in the United States, *Journal of the American Medical Association*, 270: 2207–2208.

McWilliam, E. (1996) Touchy Subjects: A Risky Enquiry into Pedagogical Pleasure, *British Educational Research Journal*, 22: 305–319.

—— (1999) *Pedagogical Pleasures*, New York: Peter Lang.

—— (2004) Getting Passionate: The Recovery of the Emotions in Educational Leadership, paper presented at the Australian Association for Research in Education Conference Doing the Public Good: Positioning Education Research, Melbourne, 28 November–2 December.

Miah, A. (2005) Genetics, Cyberspace and Bioethics: Why not a Public Engagement with Ethics?, *Public Understanding of Science*, 14: 409–421.

—— (2008) Justifying Human Enhancement: The Accumulation of Biocultural Capital, in S. Wint (ed.) *Ethical Futures: Boundaries to Human Enhancement*, London: Royal Society for the Encouragement of the Arts.

Miah, A. and Rich, E. (2008) *The Medicalisation of Cyberspace*, London and New York: Routledge.

Mills, C.W. (1959) *The Sociological Imagination*, Harmondsworth: Penguin.

Monaghan, L.F. (2005a) Big Handsome Men, Bears and Others: Virtual Construction of 'Fat Male Embodiment', *Body and Society*, 11: 81–111.

—— (2005b) Discussion Piece: A Critical Take on the Obesity Debate, *Social Theory and Health*, 3 (4): 302–314.

—— (2006a) Body Mass Index, Masculinities and Moral Worth: Men's Critical Understandings of 'Appropriate Weight for Height', *Sociology of Health and Illness*, 29 (4): 584–609.

—— (2006b) Weighty Words: Expanding and Embodying the Accounts Framework, *Social Theory and Health*, 4 (2): 128–167.

Moore, K. (1998) Anorexics' Narratives on Recovery, unpublished MA thesis, University of East Anglia.

Morais, A., Neves, I., Davies, B. and Daniels, H. (eds) (2001) *Towards a Sociology of Pedagogy: The Contribution of Basil Bernstein to Research*, New York: Peter Lang.

Moynihan, R. (2007) Expanding Definitions of Obesity May Harm Children, *BMJ* 2006. Available at: http://bmj/cgi/content/full/332/7555/1412 (accessed 6 February 2008).

Murphy, P. (1995) The Body Politic, in P.A. Komesaroff (ed.) *Troubled Bodies: Critical Perspectives on Postmodernism, Medical Ethics and the Body*, London: Duke University Press.

National Audit Office (2001) *Tackling Obesity in England: Report by the Comptroller and Auditor General*, London: Her Majesty's Stationery Office.

—— (2006) *Tackling Childhood Obesity – First Steps*, London: Her Majesty's Stationery Office.

Nettleton, S. (1992) *Power, Pain and Dentistry*, Buckingham: Open University Press.

—— (1997a) Governing the Risky Self: How to Become Healthy, Wealthy and Wise, in A. Petersen and R. Bunton (eds) *Foucault, Health and Medicine*, London: Routledge.

—— (1997b) Surveillance, Health Promotion and the Formation of a Risk Identity, in M. Sidell, L. Jones, J. Katz and A. Peberdy (eds) *Debates and Dilemmas in Promoting Health*, London: Open University Press.

Nettleton, S. and Bunton, R. (1995) Sociological Critique of Health Promotion, in R. Bunton, S. Nettleton and R. Burrows (eds) *The Sociology of Health Promotion*, London: Routledge.

Neumark-Sztainer, D. (2005) Can We Simultaneously Work Toward the Prevention of Obesity and Eating Disorders in Children and Adolescents?, *International Journal of Eating Disorders*, 38 (3): 220–227.

Noddings, N. (1992) *The Challenge to Care in Schools*, New York: Teachers College Press.

—— (2002) *Educating Moral People: A Caring Alternative to Character Education*, New York: Teachers College Press.

O'Brien, K.S., Hunter, J.A. and Banks, M. (2007) Implicit Anti-fat Bias in Physical Educators: Physical Attributes, Ideology and Socialisation, *International Journal of Obesity*, 3 (2): 308–314.

O'Dea, J.A. (2004) Prevention of Child Obesity: First, Do No Harm, *Health Education Research: Theory and Practice*, 20 (2): 259–265.

—— (2005) School-based Health Education Strategies for the Improvement of Body Image and Prevention of Eating Problems: An Overview of Safe and Effective Interventions, *Health Education*, 105 (1): 11–33.

—— (2007) *Everybody's Different: A Positive Approach to Teaching about Health, Puberty, Body Image, Self Esteem and Obesity Prevention*, Melbourne: ACER Press.

O'Dea, J.A. and Maloney, D. (2000) Prevention of Eating and Body Image Problems in Children and Adolescents Using the Health Promoting Schools Framework, *Journal of School Health*, 70 (1): 18–21.

Ofsted (2005) *Framework for the Inspection of Schools in England from September 2005*, Manchester: Ofsted.

Oliver, J. (2000) *The Return of the Naked Chef*, London: Penguin.

—— (2001) *Happy Days with the Naked Chef*, London: Michael Joseph.

—— (2003) *Funky Food for Comic Relief – Red Nose Day*, London: Penguin.

Oliver, K. (2001) Images of the Body from Popular Culture: Engaging Adolescent Girls in Critical Inquiry, *Sport, Education and Society*, 6 (2): 143–164.

Oliver, K.L. and Lalik, R. (2000) *Bodily Knowledge: Learning about Equity and Justice with Adolescent Girls*, New York: Peter Lang.

Parsons, T. (1978) *Action Theory and the Human Condition*, New York: Free Press.

—— (1991 [1951]) *The Structure of Social Action*, London: Routledge.

Penney, D. and Evans, J. (1999) *Politics, Policy and Practice in Physical Education*, London: E. and F.N. Spon.

Penney, D. and Harris, J. (2004) The Body and Health in Policy: Representations and Recontextualizations, in J. Evans, B. Davies and J. Wright (eds) *Body Knowledge and Control: Studies in the Sociology of Physical Education and Health*, London: Routledge.

Peterson, A. and Bunton, R. (eds) (1997) *Foucault, Health and Medicine*, London: Routledge.

Piran, N. (1999) The Reduction of Preoccupation with Body Weight and Shape in Schools: A Feminist Approach, in N. Piran, M.P. Levine and C. Steiner-Adair (eds) *Preventing Eating Disorders*, Philadelphia, PA: Brunner/Mazel.

—— (2004) Teachers: On 'Being' (rather than 'Doing') Prevention, *Eating Disorders*, 12: 1–9.

Platt, A. (1971) The Rise of the Child-saving Movement, in B.R. Cosin, I.R. Dale, G.M. Esland and D.F. Swift (eds) *School and Society: A Sociological Reader*, London: Routledge & Kegan Paul in association with the Open University.

Power, S. (2000) Educational Pathways into the Middle Class(es), *British Journal of Sociology of Education*, 21 (2): 133–147.

Power, S. and Whitty, G. (2002) Bernstein and the Middle Class, *British Journal of Sociology of Education*, 23 (4) (special issue: Basil Bernstein's Theory of Social Class, Educational Codes and Social Control): 595–607.

Prince, R. (1985) The Concept of Culture Bound Syndrome: Anorexia Nervosa and Brain-fag, *Social Science Medicine*, 21: 197–203.

Pronger, B. (2002) *Body Fascism: Salvation in the Technology of Physical Fitness*, Toronto: University of Toronto Press.

Prout, A. (2000) *The Body, Childhood and Society*, Basingstoke: Macmillan Press.

Puhl, R. and Brownell, K. (2001) Bias, Discrimination, and Obesity, *Obesity Research*, 9: 778–805.

Qualifications and Curriculum Authority (QCA) (2007) Physical Education: Programmes of Study for Key Stage 3 and Attainment Targets. Available at: http://curriculum.qca. org.uk/uploads/QCA-07-3342-p_PE_KS3_tcm6-407.pdf (accessed 10 October 2007).

Quennerstedt, M. (2007) Health in Physical Education – A Problem or a Possibility?, paper presented at NFPF/NERA Conference, Turkku, Finland, 15–17 March.

—— (2008) Exploring the Relation between Physical Activity and Health – A Salutogenic Approach to Physical Education, *Sport, Education and Society*, 13: in press.

Rabinow, P. and Rose, N. (2006) Biopower Today, *Biosocieties*, 1: 195–217.

Ransley, J. (1998) Eating Disorders and Adolescents: What Are the Issues for Secondary Schools?, *Health Education*, 99 (1): 35–42.

Rathner, G. (2001) Post-communism and the Marketing of the Thin Ideal, in A. Nasser, M.M. Katzman and R.A. Gordon (eds) *Eating Disorders and Cultures in Transition*, Hove: Brunner Routledge.

Rich, E. and Evans, J. (2005) Making Sense of Eating Disorders in Schools, *Discourse: Studies in the Cultural Politics of Education*, 26 (2): 247–262.

—— (forthcoming) Now I am NO-body, See Me for Who I Am: The Paradox of Performativity, *Gender and Education.*

Rich, E. and Harjunen, H. (2004) 'Normal Gone Bad' – Exploring Discourses of Health and the Female Body in Schools, paper presented at the Third Global Conference on Making Sense of Health, Illness and Disease, Oxford, July.

Rich, E., Harjunen, H. and Evans, J. (2006) 'Normal Gone Bad' – Health Discourses, Schools and the Female Body, in P. Twohig and V. Kalitzkus (eds) *Bordering Biomedicine Interdisciplinary Perspectives on Health, Illness and Disease*, Amsterdam and New York: Rodopi.

Rich, E., Holroyd, R. and Evans, J. (2004) 'Hungry to Be Noticed': Young Women, Anorexia and Schooling, in J. Evans, B. Davies and J. Wright (eds) *Body Knowledge and Control: Studies in the Sociology of Physical Education and Health*, London: Routledge.

Ritenbaugh, C. (1982) Obesity as a Culture Bound Syndrome, *Culture, Medicine and Psychiatry*, 6: 348–361.

Rogge, M.M. and Greenwald, M. (2004) Obesity, Stigma and Civilized Oppression, *Advances in Nursing Science*, 27: 301–315.

Rose, N. (1996) Governing 'Advanced' Liberal Democracies, in A. Barry, T. Osborne and N. Rose (eds) *Foucault and Political Reason: Liberalism, Neo-liberalism and Rationalities of Government*, London: UCL Press.

Routledge, P. (2007) They're Dying to Live in the North, *Daily Mirror*, 14 September.

Royal College of Physicians (2004) *Storing up Problems: The Medical Case for a Slimmer Nation*, London: RCP.

Russell-Mayhew, S. (2006) Stop the War on Weight: Obesity and Eating Disorders: Working Together toward Health, *Eating Disorders*, 14: 253–263.

Sachs, J. (2004) Watching Yourself and Others: Touch, Personal Space and Risk in the Classroom, paper presented at the Australian Association for Research in Education Conference Doing the Public Good: Positioning Education Research, Melbourne, 28 November–2 December.

Saukko, P. (1999) Fat Boys and Goody Girls: Hilde Bruch's Work on Eating Disorders and the American Anxiety about Democracy, 1930–1960, in J. Sobal and D. Maurer (eds) *Weighty Issues: Fatness and Thinness as Social Problems*, New York: Aldine De Gruyter.

Sayer, A. (2005) *The Moral Significance of Class*, Cambridge: Cambridge University Press.

Schools Health Education Unit (2003) *Trends: Young People's Food Choices, 1983–2001*, Exeter: School Health Education Unit.

Seid, R.P. (1994) Too 'Close to the Bone': The Historical Context for Women's Obsession with Slenderness, in P. Fallon, M.A. Katzman and S.C. Wooley (eds) *Feminist Perspectives on Eating Disorders*, New York: The Guilford Press.

Seidell, J.C. (2000) The Current Epidemic of Obesity, in C. Bouchard (ed.) *Physical Activity and Health*, Champaign, IL: Human Kinetics.

Shilling, C. (1993) *The Body and Social Theory*, London: Sage/TCS.

—— (2004) Educating Bodies: Schooling and the Constitution of Society, in J. Evans, B. Davies and J. Wright (eds) *Body Knowledge and Control: Studies in the Sociology of Physical Education and Health*, London: Routledge.

—— (2005) Body Pedagogics: A Programme and Paradigm for Research, paper presented to the School of Sport and Exercise Sciences, University of Loughborough.

—— (2007) *Embodying Sociology: Retrospect, Progress and Prospects*, London: Blackwell.

—— (2008) *Changing Bodies: Habit, Crisis and Creativity*, London: Sage/TCS.

Shilling, C. and Mellor, P.A. (2007) Cultures of Embodiment: Technology, Religion and Body Pedagogics, *Sociological Review*, 55 (3): 531–549.

Shore, C. and Wright, S. (1999) Audit Culture and Anthropology: Neo-liberalism in British Higher Education, *Journal of the Royal Anthropological Institute*, 5 (4): 557–575.

Skeggs, B. (1997) *Formations of Class and Gender: Becoming Respectable*, London: Sage.

Smetherham, C. (2004) First Class Women in the World of Work: Employability and Labour Market Orientations, Working Paper No. 5, Cardiff: Cardiff School of Social Sciences.

Smith, R. (2007) Don't Lose Weight after Heart Attack, *Daily Telegraph*, 10 September.

Smolak, L. and Levine, M.P. (1994) Toward an Empirical Basis for Primary Prevention of Eating Problems with Elementary School Children, *Eating Disorders: The Journal of Treatment and Prevention*, 2: 293–307.

Smolak, L., Levine, M.P. and Schermer, F. (1998) A Controlled Evaluation of an Elementary School Primary Prevention Programme for Eating Problems, *Journal of Psychosomatic Research*, 44 (3/4): 339–353.

Sobal, J. (1995) The Medicalisation and Demedicalisation of Obesity, in D. Maurer and J. Sobal (eds) *Eating Agendas: Food and Nutrition as Social Problems*, Hawthorne, NY: Aldine de Gruyter.

Sobal, J. and Maurer, D. (1999) The Social Management of Fatness and Thinness, in J. Sobal and D. Maurer, *Interpreting Weight: The Social Management of Fatness and Thinness*, New York: Aldine De Gruyter.

Solarnavigator (2008) *Jamie Oliver* (accessed 10 March 2008).

Sontag, S. (1991) *Illness as Metaphors/AIDS and its Metaphors*, London: Penguin.

Sparkes, A.C. (1995) Living Our Stories, Storying Our Lives, and the Spaces in between: Life History Research as a Force for Change, in A.C. Sparkes (ed.) *Research in Physical Education and Sport: Exploring Alternative Visions*, Lewes: Falmer Press.

Stearns, P. (1999) Children and Weight Control: Priorities in the US and France, in J. Sobal and D. Maurer (eds) *Weighty Issues: Fatness and Thinness as Social Problems*, New York: Aldine De Gruyter.

Steiner-Adair, C. and Vorenburg, A. (1999) Resisting Weightism: Media Literacy for Elementary School Children, in N. Piran, M.P. Levine and C. Steiner Adair (eds) *Preventing Eating Disorders*, Hove: Brunner/Mazel.

Stronach, I. and Corbin, B. (2002) Towards an Uncertain Politics of Professionalism: Teacher and Nurse Identities in Flux, *Journal of Education Policy*, 17: 109–138.

Sunday Times (2003) Fit or Fat: The New Class War, 8 June.

—— (2004) Talking Heads, 25 January.

Sykes, H. (2007) Anxious Identifications in 'The Sopranos' and Sport: Psychoanalytic and Queer Theories of Embodiment, *Sport, Education and Society*, 12 (2): 127–141.

Tate, A. (2000) Schooling, in B. Lask and R. Bryant-Waugh (eds) *Anorexia Nervosa and Related Eating Disorders in Childhood and Adolescence*, Hove: Psychology Press.

teachernet (2006) National Healthy Schools Standard (NHSS). Available at: http://www.teachernet.gov.uk/management/atoz/n/nhss/index.cfm?code+main (accessed 16 May 2006).

—— (2007) Supporting Healthy Lifestyles: The National Child Measurement Programme. Available at: http//www.teachernet.gov.uk/wholeschool/obesity/nationalchildmeasurementpogra (accessed 24 April 2007).

Terre Blanche, M. and Durrheim, K. (1999) Social Constructionist Methods, in M. Terre Blanche and K. Durrheim (eds) *Research in Practice: Applied Methods for the Social Sciences*, Cape Town: UCT Press.

Thompson, D. (2001) Overweight and Obesity Threaten US Health Gains, *HHS News*. Available at: http://www.sugeongeneral.gov/news/pressreleases/pr_obesity.htm (accessed 6 February 2008).

Times Magazine (2002) Fit, 19 October.

Tinning, R. (1985) Physical Education and the Cult of Slenderness, *ACPHER National Journal*, 107: 10–13.

—— (2004) Ruminations on Body Knowledge and Control and the Spaces for Hope and Happening, in J. Evans, B. Davies and J. Wright (eds) *Knowledge and Control: Studies in the Sociology of Physical Education and Health*, London: Routledge.

Treseder, P. (2007) Diet as a Social Problem: An Investigation of Children's and Young People's Perspectives on Nutrition and Body Image, unpublished Ph.D. thesis, Centre for Childhood Development and Learning, Faculty of Education and Language Studies, Open University, Milton Keynes.

Troiano, R.P., Frongillo, E.A. Jr., Sobal, J. and Levitsky, D.A. (1996) The Relationship between Body Weight and Mortality: A Quantitative Analysis of Combined Information from Existing Studies, *International Journal of Obesity*, 20: 63–75.

Turner, B.S. (1992) *Regulating Bodies: Essays in Medical Sociology*, London: Routledge.

Tyler, W. (2002) Silent, Invisible, Total: Pedagogic Discourse and the Age of Information, paper presented at the Bernstein Symposium, AARE Conference, Fremantle, Western Australia, 3–7 December.

US Department of Health and Human Services (USDHHS) (1996) *Physical Activity and Health: A Report of the Surgeon General*, Atlanta, GA: Centers for Disease Control and Prevention.

—— (2001) *The Surgeon General's Call to Action to Prevent and Decrease Overweight and Obesity*, Washington, DC: Government Printing Office.

Van Hoeken, D., Seidell, J. and Hoek, H.W. (2003) Epidemiology, in J. Treasure, U. Schmidt and E. van Furth (eds) *The Handbook of Eating Disorders*, Hoboken, NJ: John Wiley.

Wagner, T. (2007) Overweight 8 Year Old Sets off Child Obesity in Britain, *Daily Mirror*, 27 February. Available at: http://cutomwire.ap.org/dynamics/stories/B/Britain_Child _OBESITY?Site=SL (accessed 7 March 2007).

Walkerdine, V. (1990) *Schoolgirl Fictions*, London: Verso.

—— (2003) Reclassifying Upward Mobility: Femininity and the Neo-liberal Subject, *Gender and Education*, 15 (3): 237–248.

Walkerdine, V., Lucey, H. and Melody, J. (2001) *Growing up a Girl*, Basingstoke: Palgrave Macmillan.

Wallack, L. and Lawrence, R. (2005) Talking about Public Health: Developing America's 'Second Language', *American Journal of Public Health*, 95 (4): 567–570.

Walstrom, M.K. (2000) 'You Know, Who's the Thinnest?' Combating Surveillance and Creating Safety in Coping with Eating Disorders Online, *CyberPsychology and Behaviour*, 3: 761–783.

Warin, M. (2002) Becoming and Unbecoming: Abject Relations in Anorexia, unpublished Ph.D. thesis, Adelaide University.

Warin, M., Turner, K., Moore, V. and Davies, M. (2008) Bodies, Mothers and Identities: Rethinking Obesity and the BMI, *Sociology of Health and Illness*, 30 (1): 97–111.

Warmington, P., Murphy, R. and McGaig, C. (2005) Real and Imagined Crises: The Construction of Political and Media Panics over Education, *Research Intelligence*, 90: 12–13.

Watkins, C. and Mortimore, P. (1999) Pedagogy: What Do We Know?, in P. Mortimore (ed.) *Understanding Pedagogy and its Impact on Learning*, London: Sage.

Weber, M. (1991 [1904–5]) *The Protestant Ethic and the Spirit of Capitalism*, London: HarperCollins.

Weir, A. (1997) *Sacrificial Logics: Feminist Theory and the Critique of Identity*, New York: Routledge.

Wilkinson, S. (ed.) (1986) *Feminist Social Psychology: Developing Theory and Practice*, Milton Keynes: Open University Press.

Wilmott, H. (1993) Strength is Ignorance; Slavery is Freedom: Managing Culture in Modern Organisations, *Journal of Management Studies*, 30 (4): 215–252.

World Health Organisation (1998) *Obesity: Preventing and Managing the Global Epidemic: Report of a WHO Consultation on Obesity*, Geneva: WHO.

—— (2007) BMI Classification. Available at: http://www.who.int/bmi (accessed 30 October 2007).

Wright, J. and Harwood, V. (2007) Bio-power, Bio-pedagogies and the 'Obesity Epidemic', Biopedagogies Conference, Centre for Interdisciplinary Youth Research, University of Wollongong, Australia, 26–27 January.

—— (eds) (2008) *Governing Bodies: Biopolitics and the 'Obesity Epidemic'*, London: Routledge.

Wright, J., MacDonald, D. and Burrows, L. (eds) (2004) *Critical Inquiry and Problem-solving in Physical Education*, London: Routledge.

Wright, J., O' Flynn, G. and Macdonald, D. (2002) Physical Activity in the Lives of Young Women and Men: Embodied Identities, paper presented at the AISEP Conference, Coruna, Spain, 22–26 November.

—— (2006) Being Fit and Looking Healthy: Young Women's and Men's Constructions of Health and Fitness, *Sex Roles*, 54 (9–10): 707–716.

Youth Sport Trust (YST) (2002) Health on the Sports College Agenda, *TOPS, The Newsletter of the Youth Sport Trust*, 19 (spring): 1.

Zeibaland, S., Thorogood, M., Fuller, A. and Muir, J. (1996) Desire for the Body Normal: Body Image and Discrepancies between Self Reported and Measured Height and Weight in a British Population, *Journal of Epidemiology and Community Health*, 50 (1): 105–106.

Zembylas, M. (2003) Emotions and Teacher Identity: A Poststructural Perspective, *Teachers and Teaching*, 9: 213–238.

—— (2007) Risks and Pleasures: A Deleuzo-Guattarian Pedagogy of Desire in Education, *British Educational Research Journal*, 33 (4): 331–349.

Index